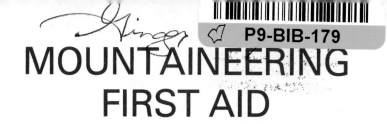

MOUNTAINEERING FIRST AID

A Guide to Accident Response and First Aid Care

Text by Dick Mitchell
Illustrations by Bruce Becker

THE MOUNTAINEERS • SEATTLE, WASHINGTON

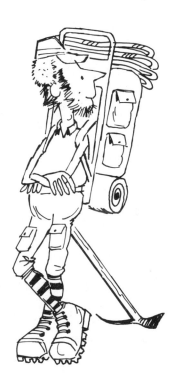

THE MOUNTAINEERS
Organized 1906

To explore and study the mountains, forests, and watercourses
    of the Northwest;
To gather into permanent form the history and traditions of this
    region;
To preserve by the encouragement of protective legislation
    or otherwise the natural beauty of Northwest America;
To make explorations into these regions in fulfillment of the above
    purposes;
To encourage a spirit of good fellowship among all lovers of
    outdoor life.

Copyright © 1972 by The Mountaineers

Second edition September 1975
Second printing, second edition, January 1977
Third printing, June 1978
Fourth printing, September 1979
Fifth printing, September 1980

Published by The Mountaineers
719 Pike Street, Seattle, Washington 98101

Published simultaneously in Canada by
Douglas & McIntyre Ltd., 1615 Venables St.
Vancouver, B.C. V5L 2H1

Manufactured in the United States of America

Library of Congress Catalog Card No. 72-94645
ISBN 0-9 16890-33-3

FOREWORD

In 1968, the Seattle Mountaineers, in cooperation with the Seattle-King County Chapter of the American Red Cross, developed a program of first aid instruction designed to meet the training requirements of those who ventured into the mountains where medical help was distant. It emphasized not only the specific first aid skills required in the event of an emergency but also the pre-trip preparation and response required at the scene of an accident should first aid or evacuation be necessary. Since its development, this program has seen a rapid growth in enrollment. The growth can be attributed to a tremendous effort by the Mountaineers, Seattle, in promoting first aid training, as well as a quality instructional program. This program is of benefit not only to the technical climber but any hiker who enjoys leisurely pursuits in unpopulated areas. It is hoped that by knowing first aid and the procedures to follow at the scene of an accident, many accidents will be prevented, and injuries reduced.

This publication is a result of experience gained from this First Aid Training Program and is designed to serve as a supplement to first aid courses in that it adapts currently established principles of first aid and emergency care to the circumstances and situations one can reasonably expect to find when venturing into the unpopulated areas. I heartily recommend that any person who enjoys outdoor pursuits or who anticipates activity in the mountains consider this type of training as one of the essentials of his equipment. In essence, first aid training should become the eleventh essential.

NORMAN G. BOTTENBERG, Director
Safety Programs
Seattle-King County Chapter
American Red Cross

TABLE OF CONTENTS

ACKNOWLEDGEMENTS

A number of individuals have contributed ideas, philosophy, and comments to this publication. Some of these are: Norm Bottenberg, Sam Fry, Larry Penberthy, Dr. Dave Rabak, Herm Gross, Dr. Les Harms, Russ Post, George Sainsbury, Wayne Misenar, Dr. Richard Birchfield, and Dr. Otto Trott. Many others, additionally, contributed either as interested individuals, authors of referenced publications, or as members of The Mountaineers, Seattle Mountain Rescue Council, American Red Cross, or National Ski Patrol. To all, thank you. The composite of your thoughts, either directly or indirectly, is reflected in this book. Special thanks, too, go to Bruce Becker for his outstanding illustrative cartoons; to Peggy Ferber for her typing, proofreading, and editorial support, and to Howard Stansbury for his encouragement and assistance.

Finally, the most important thank you goes to my family for their thoughtfulness during the hundreds of hours in which I was buried under the pages of this text.

Dick Mitchell

introduction

When an accident occurs in the mountains, response normally involves more than simply securing a bandage in place. Response involves a complex sequence of almost simultaneous actions that must be correctly and completely performed if the victim is to survive. It involves the entire accident scene, including the physical and mental states of both victim and the other party members. It involves ALL actions by the party before the accident and in response to the accident until the victim has been safely evacuated to medical facilities. As an example, part of taking care of the victim of an accident is to maintain his body warmth. This can be accomplished by isolating him from the surroundings using insulative pads, clothing or sleeping bags, and by providing heat by fire, hot liquids and food. This cannot be done, however, unless these materials are available. Unless members of the party have planned for the worst and realized the seriousness of an accident situation PRIOR to leaving home, sleeping bags, fire starters and extra food may never be included on the trip. This is why properly managing accident situations DOES NOT start after the accident occurs, but before, at home when planning what to take. It occurs before the trip when assigning rope leaders, an assistant leader, and when notifying the members of the intended route and terrain difficulty. It occurs, also, while on the climb as members continually ask themselves what they would do if an accident occurred. This book emphasizes that with adequate planning, and a realization of the tremendous problems that can occur in an accident situation, mountaineers can deal with accidents effectively and, in fact, can help in preventing them.

This book emphasizes, too, that an accident situation is one instance in which the leader, no matter how well qualified, cannot do everything himself. Each party member must contribute his share rather than doing nothing, or worse, being a hindrance to others. Proper accident response requires that the party members work closely together as a TEAM, probably relying more on one another than at any other time in mountaineering. The life of the victim, and perhaps the lives of the entire party, depend on the team's ability to think and act clearly and correctly. They cannot phone a doctor or summon an ambulance. They cannot count on outside help of any kind for many hours. That is why IT IS THE RESPONSIBILITY OF ALL WHO VENTURE INTO THE MOUNTAINS TO POSSESS A WORKING KNOWLEDGE OF HOW TO PROPERLY RESPOND TO AN ACCIDENT SITUATION.

How can one learn proper response to an accident? Just as with climbing, skiing, driving a car, or any other skill, one must learn the basics from someone qualified to teach and then PRACTICE under qualified supervision. Going into the mountains without knowing what to do is just as dangerous for the individual, and perhaps for the people around him, as driving a car without knowing how.

Throughout the United States there are a number of courses of recognized merit that teach first aid and emergency care. In some communities the American Red Cross offers a mountaineering-oriented first aid and accident response course which provides the student ACTUAL PRACTICAL EXPERIENCE at solving a number of simulated mountaineering accident problems. Such a course provides the student with the instruction and experience necessary to immediately and correctly respond to nearly any mountaineering, or community, accident situation. This text acts as a supplement.

In accomplishing the above, there are a number of things this text is not intended to do. It is just as important to understand these as it is to understand its purpose. This book, for example, is not intended as a medical reference, but, as explained above, a supplement to those taking first aid training. IT DOES NOT ATTEMPT TO COVER EVERY POSSIBILITY, BUT ONLY SUMMARIZES THE MORE COMMON PROBLEMS, WITH EMPHASIS ON LIFE-THREATENING EMERGENCIES AND MAJOR INJURIES WHICH REQUIRE IMMEDIATE ATTENTION AND CARE.

This book, additionally, is not intended to be for the sole use of the climber but rather any outdoorsman who ventures into the mountains, whether hiker, ski mountaineer, botanist, hunter, fisherman, snowmobiler, boy scout, or casual outdoor traveler who occasionally simply prefers to "get away." All of these individuals may encounter accidents in remote areas, and may need the skills taught herein.

After understanding the purpose and limitations of this publication, then, the reader is prepared to begin.

causes of accidents

In the last 20 years more people were involved in mountaineering accidents in Washington, California, Wyoming, and Colorado than all other states combined. Statistics indicate that although most of these accidents involved people with little or no mountaineering experience (two to one), those who were constantly in the mountains were far more likely to see or be involved in one. Those accidents most likely occurred on rock, rather than snow (two to one), where an individual either slipped or a rock fell on him. Rarely (less than 10% of combined incidents) was the accident caused by avalanche, medical illness, an improper rappel or improper use of belay. Evidence indicates that most accidents don't just happen—they are caused. Neglect, lack of technical knowledge or common sense, or physical or mental fatigue are all precipitating factors. Experience tells us it is far better to be prepared for an accident than to simply climb without the realization of the problems that can occur after an accident. Guidelines like the Mountaineers' " Climbing Code" (see references; *Mountaineering: The Freedom of the Hills)* assist the climber in defining safe practices, but, in the long run, do not substitute for years of experience, knowledge and mature judgment.

defining
first
aid

First aid is defined as "the immediate care given to a person who has been injured or suddenly taken ill." To you, as a first aider, this means two very important things:

1. That the first aid you perform must be IMMEDIATE. In some cases you should respond in less than a minute; in other cases you can wait several minutes before doing something. But in nearly every problem encountered in the mountains, the first aid must normally be accomplished in a relatively short time, although evacuation may be delayed for hours or days.

2. First aid is the immediate CARE given. This includes not only the bandaging of the victim's physical injuries but the caring for his entire mental and physical being. A wound is more than just bleeding. It involves pain, concern, anxiety, worry, and apprehension. All of these must be attended to by the first aider—mental and emotional as well as physical needs.

Nearly all injured people want help. They want to know they will be all right; they want reassurance. This does not mean to lie to them. It does mean that they want the assurance of knowing someone qualified is there to help. They want to know what their injuries are (approximately) and what the first aider plans to do. In short, they normally want someone to talk to. This serves the first aider's needs too since it enables him to determine how he is doing (e.g. does it hurt here?), and relieves apprehension on his part. This process, talking and attending to the victim's emotional needs is called "Tender Loving Care" (T.L.C.). It includes keeping him warm, comfortable, fed, busy, interested, happy, confident . . . and brave, carefree, and reverent, if applicable. T.L.C. is extremely important. It cannot be overemphasized.

legal
implications

There is no legal obligation to aid an injured person unless one has negligently caused the injury. (The latter case may be extended to apply to a member of the climbing party or the climb leader, if his actions or directions to the party are construed as negligent and to have caused the injury.) Nonetheless, whether there is legal obligation or not, most individuals feel a moral obligation to assist. In that case, if assistance is rendered, it must be performed in a reasonably careful manner. In legal terminology this means that one must exercise the same care an ordinarily prudent person would exercise under similar circumstances. An untrained individual would, for example, never administer drugs, attempt to set a shoulder dislocation, perform surgery, etc., even if the equipment were available and conditions were perfect. Following the letter of the law, if one has been trained only in first aid techniques, then he is bound to confine himself to performing FIRST AID—not SECOND AID, no matter how severe or justified the circumstances. As a point of interest, although a legal basis for suit may exist in circumstances where aid has been voluntarily rendered, lawsuits, resulting from inadequate or negligent care during mountaineering accidents, are unknown.

preparing for an accident

Before leaving the city

Advance preparation assists in preventing accidents and assumes that if an accident does occur, response will be rapid and effective. Such preparation is simple and generally requires only a minimum of time. The challenge, however, is to motivate oneself to prepare for something that is not expected to occur.

Preparation includes both mental and physical effort: mentally, in acquiring knowledge and in planning; physically, in terms of conditioning (discussed later) and in packing the essential equipment. To prepare mentally one must obtain a working knowledge of first aid and other specifics of the particular outdoor activity, such as belaying, pitching a tarp, selecting a campsite, etc. Adequate planning consists of choosing a leader and an assistant leader, and ensuring that they understand their responsibilities, of selecting the route, checking current weather and trail conditions, establishing turn-back and rope-up policies, reviewing the capability of the party members, notifying the appropriate agency or friends of the party's plans, and deciding what equipment and supplies to take.

When packing for an outing, enough supplies must be taken to sustain the party members under the worst possible circumstances. Each member should ALWAYS assume that an emergency bivouac may be required and pack accordingly. This does not mean that each member need carry a sleeping bag, Ensolite pad, and tent, but that each should have enough equipment to survive the night under the worst conditions during that time of year and locality. If trail hiking, for example, in a forested summer environment with a 48-hour forecast of clear and mild weather, then emergency bivouac equipment might include only a plastic tube tent (in case of rain) and some extra food and clothing. If necessary then, a shelter could be improvised, fire built, food and fluids warmed, and the party could survive. Note the word is "survive," not "enjoy the night." For anything other than pure survival, obviously, more equipment must be carried; it is the individual's choice how much discomfort he is prepared to endure.

Not only must each member prepare for the worst when packing, but he must (morally at least) prepare for the inadequacy of others. Obviously, any leader of any outing will automatically do this since it is up to him to ensure party safety. But also, it is a responsibility of each party member to toss in a little something in EXCESS of his own needs that could be given the victim of an accident. In accident situations under inclement weather conditions, sometimes there is a tendency to withhold the donation of personal equipment to the victim. Perhaps there is a feeling that the donors will need it themselves later. This, obviously, is extremely unfortunate and, therefore, each member MUST feel there are articles within his pack in EXCESS of his own needs. The victim may very well NOT have enough for himself.

There are a number of other items which should be carried when venturing into any mountain or wilderness environment. Without them, it may be extremely difficult, if not impossible, to respond adequately in an emergency situation. These **Ten Essentials of Accident Response** weigh less than 2 pounds total and are supplemental to the mountaineering ten essentials listed later in this chapter:

1. **Ground insulation** (Size, 12 x 18 x 3/8 inches; weight 1 ounce). If each member of the party carried a small piece of polyethylene foam to place under a victim, he could easily be insulated from the ground or snow. It is extremely important that this be done. Body heat loss, particularly if an accident occurs during heavy exertion, will be very rapid. At other times, the insulation can be used to sit on, placed under a stove, or leaned against during a cold bivouac.

2. **Tube shelter** (weight 5 ounces). A tube shelter is an extremely lightweight life-saving essential. In a downpour, the victim must be kept warm and dry. If his injuries permit, he must be moved into something that won't wick water or blow away.

3. **Saw** (weight 6 ounces, length 15 inches). A small trimming saw can be easily fitted vertically into almost any pack. Its uses are: a) a splint for forearm or wrist fractures, b) for cutting ice blocks in constructing an emergency igloo or snow shelter, and c) for sawing branches for an emergency fire or in constructing a branch stretcher. You can appreciate the need for a saw if you have ever tried to cut 2-inch slide alder with a pocket knife.

4. **Twine** (80 feet x 1/8 inch, hemp, weight 4 ounces). For constructing a branch stretcher, it is much better than cutting up a rope (and much less expensive). Besides, twine can be used for dozens of other applications from hanging up wet clothes to catching fish.

5. **First aid and rescue directions.** Since no one's memory is perfect, one should carry a checklist of information on what first aid to perform for various injuries or what rescue techniques should be

initiated, if any. CAUTION: If such information is used, do not do so over the victim. Nothing can reduce the confidence of an already terrified victim faster than watching the first aider reading how to splint a fractured ankle.

6. **Wire splint** (weight 4 ounces, prepackaged). This item need not be carried on all trips, but should always be considered. For example, below timberline the first aider can readily improvize a splint from a branch or stick. If the party is above timberline, however, an ice ax cannot be used to adequately splint an arm, forearm or wrist. Its use may very well cause more harm than good. In this case, a wire splint, disassembled packsack, or ice or piton hammer is essential.

7. **Thermometer** (-40 to +120 degrees F, weight 2 ounces). This item is used to determine the temperature of water prior to immersion of frostbitten fingers or toes (102 to 105 degrees F). The elbow-dunking trick may work at home for baby's bath, but don't count on it in the mountains. If you suspect an individual has a fever, check it. Although the accuracy isn't perfect, you at least will get some idea if infection, illness, or hypothermia is a problem.

8. **Flare** (weight 4 ounces, 1 ½ inch diameter x 5 inches). The possibility of helicopter evacuation is high, and a helicopter pilot needs to know the wind speed and direction. This can be indicated by using a streamer (which is difficult to see at height) or a smoke flare. U.S. Coast Guard-approved day smoke flares are extremely effective. The wooden handle can be cut off to lighten the load.

9. **Marking tape** (25 feet, weight 1 ounce). More than one life has been saved in the past few years because the individuals going for help marked their way back. Those going out for help may not return to the accident scene for any number of reasons; pinpointing the accident location on a map is often not enough. Also, if those going for help get lost, they have a method of retracing their steps.

10. **Accident form and pencil.** Thoroughly completing an accident report is absolutely essential. It serves as a checklist to ensure that everything possible has been done for the victim, and that those going for help have correct and accurate information. It allows you to collect the information for subsequent analysis while it's available and readily remembered. Later you may inaccurately guess distances, times, locations, etc.

Even better, fill out two forms. Give one to those going for help, to be forwarded to the sheriff, and the other to the party leader for future use in answering questions.

The mountaineering ten essentials include: a map of the area, a compass, and knowledge of how to use them; a flashlight with extra batteries and bulb; extra food and clothing, preferably wool; sunglasses, pocket knife; matches in a waterproof container; candle or other firestarter and practice in building a fire with wet wood; first aid kit and knowledge of how to properly use it. For complete discussion, see references — *Mountaineering: The Freedom of the Hills.*

Before leaving the trailhead

Most of the last minute preparation of the party members must be initiated and coordinated by the leader and his assistant. They should:

1. Introduce each member to the others.
2. Inform the party of the route, its dangers, technical difficulty, and timetable.
3. Explain the turn-back and rope-up policies.
4. Indicate they have a list of party members, flares, a group first aid kit, etc.
5. Identify members with first aid experience.
6. Ensure the party as a whole carries adequate and applicable equipment such as Ensolite, sleeping bags, tents, thermometer, stove and fuel, biovouac equipment and rope.

Only after these things have been done is the party ready to leave.

During the climb

Members should think as they travel of possible evacuation routes, possible anchor points and, more generally, what they would do if someone were injured. Again, that does not mean that one has to think of nothing else, but occasionally assess the situation. Occasionally rehearse mentally what would happen if . . .

general directions for accident response

When an accident occurs, there are several things that must be done — some immediately and some later. All, however, are extremely important. They are referred to as "General Directions" and apply to any type of accident. They are, IN ORDER:

1. **Take charge of the situation.** The party leader must take charge of the situation immediately, organizing and assigning specific individuals to do certain tasks. If he is injured, the assistant leader must assume command. The party must abide by his decisions without argument, although he should remain flexible enough to consider suggestions.

2. **Approach the victim safely.** Approach to the victim must be rapid but safe. It is important not only to protect the victim from further harm caused by rockfall, avalanche, or falling rescuers, but to protect the rest of the party as well. If the terrain is steep, difficult, or hazardous, keep the rest of the party back. Have them begin to prepare a shelter, pool equipment, build a fire, etc., as one or two of the best qualified personnel approach the victim. These persons should be prepared with the proper equipment, including first aid kits, extra food and water, clothing, slings, carabiners, ropes, Ensolite, etc., particularly if the victim is perched precariously on a ledge or in an otherwise difficult position. Approach should be from the side or even below, if possible, rather than from directly above.

3. **Perform urgently needed first aid and emergency rescue.** If the victim is injured in an area of high potential snow or rock avalanche or extreme lightning danger, move him quickly to a safer location, but DO NOT cause further injury. Check, as a minimum, to see if he is breathing, has a pulse, or is severely bleeding. These checks take only a few seconds and allow the rescuer to assess the relative physical hazard versus the need to provide the victim life-saving first aid. In a few isolated instances,

16

immediate rescue may be the most urgent care the aider can provide.

Check for breathing quickly by placing your ear to the victim's nose to listen for and feel an air exchange. Simultaneously, watch for and feel rise and fall of the chest. If the victim is not breathing, begin artificial respiration. Check, then, to determine if the victim has a pulse, and, if not, initiate cardiopulmonary resuscitation. Run your hands rapidly over all body parts to detect blood. If bleeding is detected, rip away the clothes so that the wound can be examined, and immediately apply direct pressure to control it. Waste no time. LOUDLY request assistance if needed.

4. **Treat for shock.** Whatever the extent of the injuries, the victim will require warmth, rest, and fluids. Therefore, keep him lying down and insulated from the ground with Ensolite, ropes, packs, clothing, etc. Cover him with clothing and tarps to maintain his body warmth and conserve his energy. Administer a warm salted solution if he desires it. REMEMBER: Use the victim's belongings FIRST; you may need your own later.

5. **Check for other injuries.** Once the life-threatening emergencies have been identified and controlled, the victim can be examined in more detail. Be extremely thorough. At this point, there is no hurry. Start with the head. Feel all areas to locate bleeding, deformity, tenderness or pain. Examine the ears and nose for evidence of spinal fluid or blood. Feel each cervical vertebra to see if it is intact. Determine if the pupils react normally to light and if they can track movement. Ask the victim questions to determine if he is fully aware of his surroundings, whether he has lost consciousness or whether he can add one digit numbers. Examine his mouth, especially the inside to determine if there is any injury to the jaw, teeth, gums or tongue. Feel the victim's mouth, nose and ears to ensure there is no underlying injury. Continue in the same thorough manner until all injuries are identified everywhere on the body.

6. **Plan what to do.** After urgently needed first aid has been given, the victim is warm and as comfortable as possible, and all injuries are known, then time can be spent planning what else to do and how it should be done. It must be decided whether the victim be allowed to walk under his own power or should be evacuated by the party. The leader must determine if outside help is needed. (The recommendation here is that even for minor injuries, if there is uncertainty as to the victim's condition, party strength and capability, etc., outside help should be summoned.) Should the victim remain where he is until outside help arrives or should he be moved a short distance to a more sheltered area? Additionally, the leader needs to reassess what equipment and supplies are

Sequence of first aid treatment

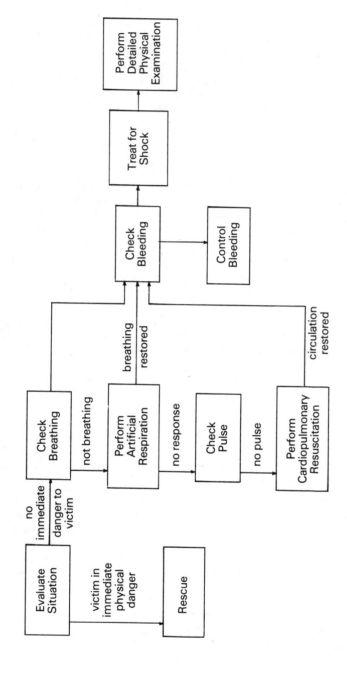

available to perform further first aid, provide for shelter and to assist in the evacuation. He must evaluate the victim's injuries, party size and physical condition, the terrain, weather, party's location with respect to outside assistance, time of day and season of year, etc. In short, the situation needs a cool analysis and development of a comprehensive plan of action.

7. **Carry out the indicated plan.** After a complete examination of the entire accident situation, the party is ready to carry out its plans. There are a number of things that may need to be done:

   a. Gather and prepare the information required by those going for help.
   b. Prepare shelters for the victim and the rest of the party.
   c. Gather wood for fires and for splinting.
   d. Prepare hot food and drink for the victim, party, and subsequent rescue personnel.
   e. Clear a helicopter landing zone.
   f. Prepare a stretcher for the victim.
   g. Set up appropriate belays and lowering equipment.
   h. Clear the trail ahead for later evacuation.
   i. Inventory available equipment and supplies.

   It is important that these not only be done for the victim, but for the rest of the party as well. Their welfare must always be considered. They too can suffer from "shock" (psychological) by simply seeing and being involved in the accident, severe bleeding, or death. This psychological condition can be just as deadly as an avalanche sweeping over the party. Often party members will become very despondent and not only unable to help in the rescue situation but highly susceptible to accidents themselves. Such problems should be treated BEFORE they occur. The party MUST be kept busy productively preparing for a successful evacuation.

It may be necessary to send for help. In mountaineering situations, it will take outside help between 6 and 24 hours to arrive on the scene of an accident. If it has been determined that help is needed, a minimum of two should be sent. They should be stronger members of the party, and should flag or otherwise mark their trail out. They should have the following information:

   a. Where, when and how the accident occurred.
   b. The number of casualties, the nature and seriousness of injuries.
   c. The first aid administered at the scene, the condition of the victim, and what first aid supplies are available.
   d. Distance from the road and the type of terrain and thus the probable difficulty of evacuation.
   e. How many people and what equipment are still at the scene, and what is the party's strength.

f. If the climbing party will wait at the spot or will move to safer or more readily accessible ground.

g. What method of evacuation will be necessary—carrying by rigid stretcher, sliding on snow, lowering down steep cliffs.

h. Where the messengers are telephoning from, and where they can meet the rescue party.

i. Names and addresses of all members in the party.

Since it is extremely difficult to remember all the information required, it is most beneficial to carry some type of accident report form to serve as a checklist (a sample is shown on following pages). Those sent for help should be informed that in all areas except National Parks, call the OPERATOR and ask for the local sheriff. In National Parks, notify the nearest Park Ranger.

Accident report form

This form is to be completed in duplicate AT the scene of the accident or each injured member of the party. One form should be sent with those going for help and the other form retained by the leader.

ACCIDENT	Date:		Time:	AM ( )	PM ( )

LOCATION	Quadrangle:	Section:
	Exact Location (included marked map):	
	Terrain: Glacier ( ) Snow ( ) Brush ( ) Timber ( ) Rock ( ) Trail ( ) Heather ( ) Easy ( ) Moderate ( ) Steep ( ) Other:	

COMPLETE DESCRIP-TION OF ACCIDENT		Ascending ( ) Descending ( ) Roped ( ) Unroped ( ) Rock Fall ( ) Ice Fall ( ) Avalanche ( ) Illness ( ) Excess Heat ( ) Cold ( ) Equipment Failure ( )
	Witnesses:	Other:

INJURED PERSON	Name:		Age:	
	Address:		Male ( ) Female ( )	
	Phone:			
	Whom to Notify:	Relation:	Phone:	

INJURIES	Overall Condi-tion	Good ( ) Fair ( ) Serious ( ) Fatal ( )
		Unconscious: Yes ( ) No ( ) If yes, length of time:
		Pulse: Respiration: Temperature:
	Injury 1	Location on Body: Type of Injury:
	Injury 2	Location on Body: Type of Injury:
	Other Injuries	Location on Body: Types of Injury:

FIRST AID TREAT-MENT	General:	Bleeding Stopped ( ) Shelter Built ( ) Artificial Respiration ( ) Warm Fluids Given ( ) Treated for Shock ( ) Evacuation ( )
	Injury 1	
	Injury 2	
	Other Injuries:	

ON-THE-SCENE PLANS	Will stay put ( ) Will evacuate to trail ( ) to Road ( ) Will evacuate a short distance to shelter ( ) Will send some members out ( ) Other:
PERSONNEL	Beginners ( ) Intermediates ( ) Advanced ( ) Number: Capability for a bivouac: Yes ( ) No ( )
	ATTACH the pre-trip prepared LIST OF PARTY MEMBERS including names, addresses and phone numbers to the ACCIDENT FORM BEING TAKEN OUT.
EQUIPMENT AVAILABLE	Tents ( ) Sleeping Bags ( ) Ensolite ( ) Flares ( ) Saw ( ) Hardware ( ) Stove and Fuel ( ) Ropes ( ) Other:
WEATHER	Warm ( ) Moderate ( ) Freezing ( ) Snow ( ) Wind ( ) Sun ( ) Clouds ( ) Fog ( ) Rain ( ) Other:
TYPE OF EVACUATION RECOMND'D.	Lowering Operation ( ) Carry-out ( ) Helicopter ( ) Rigid stretcher ( ) None until specialized medical assistance ( ) Specify:
PARTY LEADER	Name:
MESSENGERS SENT FOR HELP	Names:
FURTHER INFORMA- TION, IF ANY.	
RECOMMEN- DATIONS FOR FUTURE OUTINGS	Equipment: Leadership: Route: Abilities:

artificial respiration

In the mountains, the normal process of breathing may be interrupted by a number of factors. Examples include: lightning (electric shock); crushing or suffocation by ice blocks, snow or rock; choking or strangulation by rope, clothing, packstraps, etc.; falls or blows on the head; inadequate ventilation during cooking in snow caves, igloos or tents; heart attacks; apoplexy (stroke); or drugs such as morphine, opium, barbiturates or alcohol. Whatever the cause, oxygen must be supplied immediately to the victim until the normal breathing process can resume. If some form of artificial respiration is not begun within 6 minutes, the victim will most likely die. Once artificial respiration is begun, normal breathing will usually start again within 15 minutes except in cases of electric shock, drug poisoning, or carbon monoxide poisoning. In these instances, nerves and muscles controlling the breathing system are paralyzed, deeply depressed, or in the case of carbon monoxide poisoning, the carbon monoxide has displaced oxygen in the bloodstream. When these instances are encountered, therefore, artificial respiration must often be continued for long periods. In all cases, DO NOT give up, but continue until the victim begins to breathe for himself or until the situation becomes clearly hopeless.

Advantages of mouth-to-mouth artificial respiration

The mouth-to-mouth method of artificial respiration is superior, by far, for the following reasons:

1. One person alone can provide oxygen to the victim immediately.
2. Ventilation can be obtained under almost any circumstances; e.g., with the victim partially buried in snow.
3. The rescuer can determine if an adequate exchange of air is taking place.
4. The method is not excessively fatiguing.
5. It is the most versatile technique; i.e., either mouth-to-mouth or mouth-to-nose can be administered.
6. It permits the person administering it to have his hands free to maintain an air way or to press excess air out of the victim's stomach.

23

When mouth-to-mouth artificial respiration should be performed

If the individual is having difficulty in breathing, or is not breathing at all, immediately tilt the head backward and extend the jaw forward (jutting out), thereby clearing the airway. This may be sufficient to restore normal breathing. If it does not, the victim's breathing efforts may be assisted by mouth-to-mouth or mouth-to-nose artificial respiration techniques. Breathing difficulty is evidenced by:

1. The victim is struggling to move air in and out of his lungs, or the muscles on the front of his neck stand out prominently but no air can be heard or felt moving in and out of the mouth or nose.
2. The victim's breathing is very noisy or has a bubbling sound.
3. The victim is breathing very slowly.
4. Cyanosis is present. (Cyanosis is a grayish-blue discoloration of the skin around the lips, ears, fingernails, and sometimes the whole body; it indicates a lack of oxygen.)

If the individual is NOT breathing, this can be determined by placing your ear next to the victim's nose or mouth, listening and feeling for air exchange. Simultaneously, place your hand on the victim's diaphragm (upper abdomen) to feel any movement. Feel under the clothing, not through it.

How mouth-to-mouth artificial respiration should be performed

If no sign of breathing can be detected, perform mouth-to-mouth respiration as follows:

1. Make sure the victim's head is properly positioned, with the neck extended and head tilted backward to open the airway. To do this, place the heel of one hand on the victim's forehead and the other hand under his neck. Lift the neck with one hand while tilting the head back with pressure on the forehead with the other. This

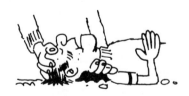

TILT HEAD BACK

usually opens the mouth automatically. Care should be taken to avoid a forceful tilting of the head of an infant, or of an unconscious victim since you could cause or there may already be a neck injury.

2. Pinch the victim's nose closed for mouth-to-mouth, or seal the victim's mouth by holding the lips together for mouth-to-nose.
3. Take a deep breath.
4. Make a tight seal with your mouth around the victim's mouth.
5. Blow air into his mouth until you see his chest expand.
6. Remove your mouth from his mouth to allow the air in his lungs to exhaust passively. Rotate your head toward his chest as you take another breath. Remember, when you see the victim's chest rise adequately, stop inflation, raise your mouth and let him exhale. Repeat this cycle 12 times a minute (once every 5 seconds). The rhythm is not as important as the volume of air blown into the lungs. The lungs must expand; this is why you must blow in until you see the chest rise.

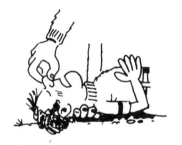

PINCH NOSE CLOSED

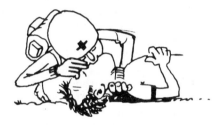

FORM AIRTIGHT SEAL
AND BLOW

7. If air is not being exchanged, open and inspect the victim's mouth. Remove any obvious obstructions and again attempt artificial respiration. If air still cannot be exchanged, quickly turn the victim on his side and administer several sharp blows between the shoulder blades to dislodge the foreign matter. Again ensure that there are no foreign objects in the throat, and that the head and jaw position are correct.

In the mouth-to-mouth technique air is easily blown into the victim's stomach if excessive force is used to fill the lungs. A stomach full of air may make lung ventilation more difficult because it pushes up on the diaphragm and increases the likelihood of vomiting. When the victim's stomach bulges, press on the stomach area with a hand to force the air out. This may also cause vomiting of the stomach contents, so turn the victim's head to one side and be prepared to clear the mouth of vomitus.

cardiopulmonary resuscitation

Artificial respiration is only of value if breathing alone will revive the victim. It is of no use if the victim's heart has stopped, since without circulation, oxygen cannot be carried to the vital organs. In that case, the action of the heart must be augmented by external compression, which, together with artificial respiration, is referred to as cardiopulmonary resuscitation (CPR). Its usage, however, although lifesaving, can be hazardous. Whereas a victim's weak breathing may be aided by mouth-to-mouth artificial respiration, if his heart is pumping, he will NOT benefit from attempts to assist his heart by compression.

To be successful, cardiopulmonary resuscitation depends on thorough and careful training. Injury is much more likely when performed by an untrained individual. Fractures of the ribs caused by improper compressions can cause injury to internal organs such as the heart, liver, or lungs. It is doubtful that one will be able to achieve artificial blood circulation by this method if his only training is from reading written instructions. For this reason, training by qualified personnel is highly recommended.

A person whose circulation has ceased because of cardiac arrest will exhibit certain signs of this condition. These are:

1. **Unconsciousness.** This will have occurred by the time that cardiac arrest would be suspected.

2. **The pulse will be absent.** The pulse in the wrist is often difficult to find even in a well person. Therefore, it should not be relied upon in determining the need for cardiopulmonary resuscitation. The strongest pulse in the body can be felt in the neck on either side of the windpipe (trachea). This is the carotid artery and this location is only a few inches from the heart. Pulses may also be felt over the brachial artery on the inner side of the upper arm and from the femoral artery in the groin. If the heart is beating, a pulse can ordinarily be felt at one or more of these locations. CAUTION: be sure you are not feeling your own pulse. It may become noticeable in your fingertips and feel very much like a weak pulse in the victim. With practice it is not difficult to distinguish your own pulse by the following maneuver. Simultaneously locate your pulse with the other hand at any of the usual locations and see if the two pulses are beating at exactly the same rate. (The individual beats will not

be felt at exactly the same instant if there is a difference in distance from the heart.)

3. **The victim will not be breathing.** (He may gasp irregularly a number of times before respiratory effort ceases.) The best place to watch for shallow breathing is the upper abdomen. Since in most conditions the heart may continue to beat for a time after breathing has stopped, absence of breathing **should not be accepted as the sole reason for heart resuscitation.**

4. **Cyanosis.** All or some of the areas that are normally pink—ear lobes, lips, tongue and finger nails—will show evidence of poor or absent oxygenation of blood during the first minute. However, if the victim normally is pallid or dark, it may not show up well.

5. **The pupils of the eyes will enlarge or dilate considerably and remain dilated.** They are an effective indicator of severe oxygen deficiency of the brain. In cardiac arrest, the pupils not only become very large, but they are unresponsive, just as in death.

The first aider must be aware of these signs and use them as indicators in determining when to start CPR and its effectiveness.

If the first aider suspects cardiac arrest, he should proceed as follows:

1. Open the airway by tilting the head back and determine if the victim is breathing. If he is not, ventilate with four quick full breaths without allowing time for the lungs to deflate completely.

2. With the tips of the index and middle fingers, determine if the victim has a carotid pulse. If a pulse is felt, continue mouth-to-mouth artificial respiration until natural breathing is restored.

3. If no pulse can be felt, initiate CPR. REMEMBER: TIME IS OF THE ESSENCE. DO NOT continue to examine the victim, seek distant assistance, remove clothing, or check the pupils. BEGIN CPR AT ONCE.

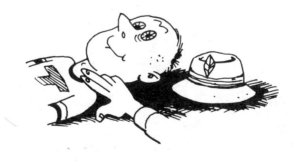

CHECK CAROTID PULSE

4. Quickly place the victim on a firm surface, face up.

5. Assume a kneeling position close to the side of the victim's chest.

6. Place the heel of one hand over the lower half of the victim's breastbone (sternum) approximately 2 inches from its lower tip. The fingers should be positioned over the victim's ribs but not touching them. The other hand should be placed on top of the first with fingers interlocked. Care must be exercised to ensure no force is applied directly over the tip of the sternum.

7. Bring the shoulders directly over the victim's sternum, keeping the arms straight (elbows locked) so that the force of compression can be applied with the weight of the upper part of the body.

8. Rocking back and forth slightly from the hip joints, exert sufficient vertically downward pressure to depress the lower sternum 1 ½ to 2 inches. Avoid sudden or jerking movements. Compressions should be smooth, regular, and uninterrupted.

9. Between strokes, the pressure must be completely relaxed to permit filling of the heart, but the rescuer's hand should remain in contact with the chest wall.

10. Apply downward pressure at the rate of 80 per minute for one rescuer and 60 per minute if two rescuers are working (one compressing and one ventilating).

DEPRESS LOWER STERNUM

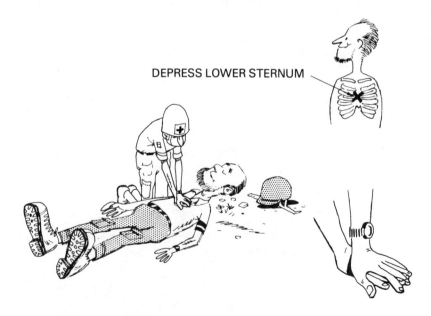

11. Synchronize lung inflation with chest compression as follows: **If the rescuer is alone:** give 15 seconds of compressions at the rate of 80 per minute then two quick lung inflations. Continue to alternate inflations and compressions — 15 compressions, 2 inflations, 15, 2, 15, 2 . . .

    If two rescuers are present: one rescuer applies chest compressions without interruption at about one compression per second (60 per minute). The other rescuer inflates the victim's lungs after every fifth chest compression. He should begin to blow as soon as the compressor starts to release pressure on the chest — 5 compressions, 1 inflation, 5, 1, 5, 1 . . . Ventilation and compression phases should be coordinated so that no interruption of chest compressions occurs.

12. Check for the effectiveness of resuscitation.
    a. The chest should visibly rise with each breath administered.
    b. If chest compression produces a detectible pulse at any of the pressure points, circulation of blood is being accomplished. This should be verified after the first minute of CPR and every few minutes thereafter. Additionally, a check every few minutes should be made to see if the victim's natural heartbeat has resumed. This is done by momentarily checking for a pulse while the chest is not being compressed. DO NOT interrupt CPR for more than 5 seconds, however.
    c. Proof that both lung ventilation AND blood circulation are being accomplished is constriction of the pupils to a more normal size. This indicates that the brain is getting oxygen. Again, this check should be made every few minutes.

13. If the victim's natural pulse has resumed, stop doing chest compressions but continue lung ventilations. When he starts trying to breathe again, coordinate mouth-to-mouth respirations with the victim's efforts, assisting rather than opposing him.

14. Continue compression as long as needed, until professional medical personnel dictate otherwise, or until absolutely certain that death has occurred. (Doctors at Johns Hopkins Medical Institute have revived victims after 105 minutes of cardiopulmonary resuscitation.)

15. Recognize that some cases of cardiac arrest cannot be resuscitated — even if you start immediately and perform CPR correctly, adequately and without interruption. A massive heart attack, severe depression from drugs or carbon monoxide, prolonged submersion in water, serious electric shock or profound asphyxia may prevent recovery despite your efforts. Recognize this fact and neither blame yourself nor become discouraged if you fail despite quick and correct application of this technique.

wounds

There are various kinds of wounds but they are all defined the same way: "a break in the surface of the skin." In mountaineering they occur in a number of ways: improper use of an ice ax, crampons, or knife, slipping or falling, exploding of a gas stove, etc. Whatever the cause, the first aid is to control bleeding and prevent contamination.

Major wounds

Major wounds can cause arterial bleeding, which occurs in pulses or spurts of bright red blood. Since arterial bleeding can be fatal in minutes, quick, decisive action is mandatory. The following steps should be taken to control any major hemorrhage:

1. Immediately apply DIRECT PRESSURE to the bleeding area! DO NOT allow severe bleeding to continue while rummaging through packs for sterile dressings; use your bare hand if necessary. When a sterile compress is available, place it directly over the wound. If bleeding continues, place additional sterile compresses on top of the old ones and continue to apply direct pressure. This stops the bleeding in nearly all instances.
2. If feasible, elevate the bleeding area. Use pressure points.
3. Apply cold packs, if available.
4. If these measures fail, and the wound is on a limb, and **only if the bleeding is severe and life-threatening,** apply a tourniquet. Apply it tightly enough to completely stop the bleeding, and once the tourniquet is in place, leave it on; do not loosen it. Tag or otherwise mark the victim to identify that a tourniquet has been placed, the time of placement, and by whom. **Remember that a decision to apply a tourniquet is essentially a decision to sacrifice that limb to save the life,** particularly in a mountaineering situation where needed help is hours away. Many physicians believe that the use of a tourniquet is PRACTICALLY NEVER JUSTIFIED.

Another type of major wound involves a large gash or tearing of the skin and underlying tissues, exposing the internal organs. These organs may even protrude through the opening, accompanied by or without severe bleeding. In these cases, if the organs are protruding, do not attempt to push them back. Keep them moist with a saline solution of 1 teaspoon of salt or 12 salt tablets in a quart of clean, preferably sterile, water. To sterilize, boil the water for 15 minutes. Cover with a number of sterile dressings and lightly bandage without excessive pressure unless necessary to control bleeding. A plastic or cellophane cover over the bandage will prevent evaporation.

Minor wounds

For minor wounds where bleeding is not a severe problem or, for the most part, has been controlled, the wound should be cleaned and dressed under as sterile conditions as possible. The method by which this is done varies depending upon the type of wound. If the wound is, for example, an **abrasion** or **avulsion** (removal of tissue), the area should be thoroughly washed, covered with sterile dressings, and bandaged. For a **puncture** wound, an even more thorough and adequate cleansing is required. The first aider should leave all but minor objects imbedded in the wound rather than risk possible further injury and bleeding by their removal. (The only exception to this is, of course, if the object would interfere with or cause further injury during evacuation.) For **lacerations** or **incisions**, the following procedure should be followed when time and weather conditions allow:

1. Wash your hands.
2. Wash the wound with a sterile compress and antibacterial soap. Always clean the wound first then work outward several inches on all sides in a circular motion, gradually increasing the diameter, rather than back and forth, Rinsing may be accomplished by irrigating with clear running water. Blot the wound dry with sterile gauze pads or a clean cloth. If the wound is surrounded by hair, shave the area 1 to 2 inches on all sides away from the wound.
3. If the wound is open, it should be closed with butterfly bandages. A butterfly can be constructed from adhesive tape as shown below:

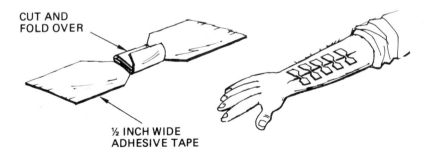

CUT AND FOLD OVER

½ INCH WIDE ADHESIVE TAPE

Apply the butterfly on one side of the wound, closing the wound with the fingers before allowing the other side of the butterfly to adhere. If the skin is cold and wet, and the adhesive quality of the tape is dubious, apply tincture of benzoin to the area around the wound. DO NOT apply tincture of benzoin to the wound itself; it is used only as an adhesive to ensure butterflies will hold. Allow the benzoin to dry before applying the butterflies. Wounds of the scalp may be closed without the aid of butterflies by tying opposing strands of hair together. Use double square knots, however, since the hair has a very stubborn tendency to untie.

4. Cover with a sterile dressing and bandage. The bandage material may be of several kinds but a roller gauze holding the sterile dressings in place covered with a triangular bandage for additional protection is the most effective. An elastic bandage also can be used, but ONLY with enough tension to secure the dressing and NO MORE. Other uses of an elastic bandage are DISCOURAGED; the danger of impeding circulation is too great.

5. Iodine, merthiolate, mercurochrome and other antiseptic solutions should not be applied directly to the wound, since they can cause tissue damage and, in the case of iodine, pain.

Even though a large amount of blood has not been lost as a result of a wound, the victim may need to be carried out. Consider if the victim were allowed to walk, whether the wound would start to bleed again, possibly with increased intensity, or enlarge by tearing.

Infection

Since the signs of infection do not appear immediately after an injury, but usually take from 2 to 7 days, infections are seldom encountered in mountaineering situations unless there has been a previous injury or the party is away from medical help for an extended period of time.

Protecting the wound from contamination and thus preventing infection, however, is of prime importance. A great deal of care and thoroughness should be exercised when cleansing even minor wounds and applying the dressings. No attempt should be made to cleanse major bleeding wounds.

shock

Shock is a depressed condition of many vital bodily functions due to the failure of sufficient blood to circulate through the body following severe injury. It can be caused by fractures, internal or external loss of FLUIDS or any significant injury combined with cold and/or pain. (Note the use of the word "fluids." This may include blood, plasma, or perspiration.) Whatever the cause, circulatory failure predisposes an individual to shock when injury occurs.

Shock SHOULD BE EXPECTED after any major injury and even after minor injuries if the victim's mental or physical condition is questionable, as in cases involving bad weather, difficult terrain, poor physical condition, etc. There are, essentially, four elements in the first aid for shock:

1. **Position.** Have the victim lie down to reduce the effort required by his heart, and to increase the warming ability of his blood circulation. Raise his feet for lower extremity wounds to increase blood volume to vital body organs, EXCEPT in cases where, additionally, there is a head injury, breathing difficulty, an unsplinted fractured lower extremity, or if the victim complains of pain when elevation is attempted. Raise the head or upper body if the victim is breathing with difficulty unless there are suspected neck or spinal injuries, if the victim complains of pain when attempted, or if there is bleeding or vomitus from the mouth (in which case turn the head sideways).

2. **Maintenance of body heat.** The amount of heat the body produces as a result of just existing, i.e., the muscles involuntarily contracting and relaxing, food digesting, etc., is called the basal metabolic rate (BMR) and equals approximately 1870 kilocalories per day. This varies, depending on a person's weight, physical condition, age, and sex. When one does deliberate physical exercise at a moderate rate (hiking up a trail with a pack), the amount of heat the body produces is approximately six times the basal metabolic rate. For heavy exertion the body produces heat equivalent to 10 times the BMR. Even shivering generates the amount of heat equivalent to running at a slow pace.

   What does this mean? After an accident, with the victim lying down, the amount of heat produced by the body drops drastically. Blood is not being circulated rapidly, and therefore, the victim cannot keep warm. To help prevent and control shock, body heat must be maintained. The victim must be insulated from the surroundings and, in some cases, warmed by application of heat. There are several ways this should be done.

a. **Insulate the victim from the ground** with Ensolite, ropes, clothing, packs, an air mattress, tree boughs, or anything else available. Even without snow, the ground is usually much cooler than the surrounding air. Too, since the thermal conductivity of water is 24 times greater than that of dry air, it is imperative that the victim be kept dry and well insulated. If he is allowed to become wet, or to remain wet, heat will be lost very rapidly, and the victim's condition will quickly deteriorate. Remove wet clothing and replace with dry garments.

b. **Cover the victim from the top** with dry insulation. Top it off with a layer of wind protective garments or sheets to avoid heat loss by conduction. Do not forget to cover the head and neck areas. Nearly 50% of the heat lost by the body is lost through the head and neck, if unprotected, at 40°F, and nearly 75% at 5°F. This is extremely important. Circulation to the head, unlike the other extremities, is not reduced in cold weather but continues to supply a constant level of oxygen to the brain.

c. **Insulate the victim from the weather** with a tent, snow cave, tarp, igloo or other improvised shelter. A well-coordinated first aid team will slip insulation under the victim while simultaneously inserting him into a collapsed tent (which can be erected later).

d. **Provide external warmth** to the victim when circumstances warrant it. CAUTION: use the utmost care to prevent a burn. Test warm objects THOROUGHLY. Rotate them to other body areas periodically. A victim in shock may not be able to adequately determine if objects are too hot. Some items that can be used are: **warm liquids or foods, a prewarmed sleeping bag, another person, warmed water bottles or rocks wrapped in clothing, or fires on either side of the victim.**

3. **Fluids.** A warm salt solution (six tablets per quart of water) should be administered to the victim slowly in small doses. The use of bouillion, tea, etc., may make the solution more palatable.

NOTE: when administering salt, either dissolve the tablets in a solution or allow the victim to take singly only wax-impregnated tablets. Although these take more time to dissolve, there is less danger of the victim becoming nauseous.

4. **Tender loving care.** As mentioned previously, this factor is a vital portion of the treatment of shock.

fractures

Fractures may be either open or closed: "open" refers to fractures in which the broken ends are protruding through the skin (also called compound fractures), and "closed" refers to fractures with no break in the skin. The first aid for either is essentially the same: dress as necessary for open wounds and splint above and below the fracture, keeping the adjacent joints quiet. This means that with a suspected fracture of the lower leg, the splint should extend above the knee and below the ankle. For a suspected fracture above the knee, a full leg splint extending from the armpit to the heel is required. Because of the prevalence of fractures in mountaineering situations, it is exceptionally important that the first aider know exactly what to do and how to do it. Consider a simple fracture of forearm or wrist. The objective is to splint the forearm using wire mesh, a piton hammer, Ensolite, branches, tent stakes, or other suitable material. The forearm should then be secured to the chest with a triangular bandage or webbing. Obviously, improvisation is the key, using webbing, tape, rope, or twine to secure the splint and forearm. In much more detail, the injury (and the victim) should be handled in the following manner.

Fracture of the forearm or wrist

1. Examine the victim EVERYWHERE for severe bleeding, thereby identifying any open fractures.
2. Finding none, proceed to the location of pain, but DO NOT touch it directly. Work to the area slowly checking for deformity, bruising, bumps, or other irregularities. Compare the suspected fractured area with another body member. Ask the victim if he heard a breaking sound, how he fell, does he suspect it is broken, etc.
3. Check other body parts AND ask victim if he hurts elsewhere.
4. Be planning ahead, thinking of the kind of splint to apply and type of material to be used.
5. "Splint them where they lie."
   a. Choose an appropriate splinting material (wire splint, branches, piton hammer).
   b. Make it the right size, if needed.
   c. Pad it with clothing, webbing, Ensolite, etc. Note: avoid the use of rubberized or plastic materials when possible. If they are placed next to the skin, the area becomes very hot, moist, and uncomfortable.

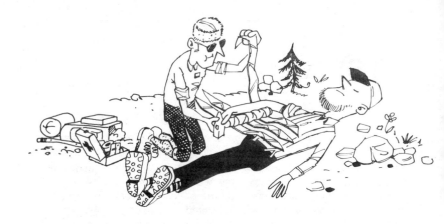

d. Place the splinting material to one side of the fracture (NOT on top of it).
e. Gently thread webbing, triangular bandages or cravats (narrow strips of cloth) under the arm, being careful not to disturb it. CAUTION: DO NOT use an elastic bandage for securing the splinting materials in place.
f. Tie the knots in an accessible place but not directly over the injury.
g. If you have to remove clothing, cut along a seam.
h. Don't hurry. Talk to victim. Ask if it is too tight. Observe any change in the color of the extremity.

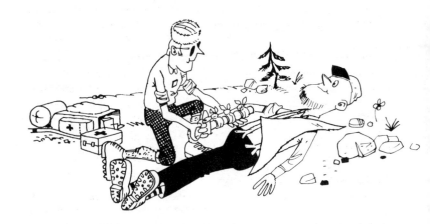

i. If the fracture involves the wrist, hand, or fingers, remove rings, watch, or bracelet before swelling makes removal difficult.
6. Prepare triangular bandage across victim's chest.
7. Move splinted forearm across chest, checking tightness of cravats.
8. Secure the triangular bandage, pad knot, and place it to one side of the neck.
9. Elevate wrist approximately 4 inches from tip of elbow.
10. Pin or tie elbow portion of triangular so that elbow will not slip out.
11. Secure the triangular to the chest using a wide cravat extending from the tip of the elbow diagonally across to the opposite shoulder.
12. Make sure fingertips are accessible (uncovered, weather permitting) to check circulation. Check frequently during transportation.
13. Treat for shock by keeping the victim lying down, warm, head and chest slightly elevated.
14. If the victim is not cold or wet, a plastic bag full of snow can be gently placed over the fracture site, thereby reducing swelling and pain.

Finger fractures

Many of the same basic principles applied when splinting a forearm are followed when splinting a finger; e.g., check for proper circulation, pad the splint, etc. For splinting material, a piton, a small branch, or rolled clothing and an adjacent finger can be used. The padded splint should be securely bound to the finger with roller gauze and then two or more fingers tied to each other. Care should be taken to immobilize the finger(s) in a natural position (called a "position of function") rather than splinting them rigidly flat. Placing the entire arm in a triangular bandage is then recommended to maintain elevation and ensure the fracture is not disturbed.

Fracture of the upper arm (humerus)

The injured arm should be placed, if pain permits, in a natural position with the elbow at right angles. Support the forearm in a sling. Apply a well padded splint on the outside of the arm, extending from the shoulder to the elbow. Tie the splint to the upper arm and secure around the body above and below the fracture. Check the color of the fingers frequently to determine if circulation is adequate.

Fracture of the elbow

Do not attempt to move the arm at the elbow joint unless absolutely necessary for transportation. If it is straight, splint it in that position by extending the splint from the fingertips to the armpit. Place the splint on the palm side (inside) of the arm. If the elbow is bent, extend the splint from the shoulder to the wrist on the outside of the arm.

Collarbone (clavicle) fractures

The normal first aid procedure for a fracture of the collarbone is to support the upper extremity on the injured side with an arm sling. A cravat is then tied around the chest to keep the arm (and thus the shoulder) from moving, and to avoid forward flexation. A means of supplementing this procedure is the use of a triangular bandage which directly pulls the shoulders back. It is secured in place before the arm sling as follows: place the middle of the triangular, point down, on the back of the neck. Pass each of the ends nearest the shoulders over them and under the armpits. Securely tie the ends at mid back. Roll and tuck in the remaining end. The proper first aid sequence is shown in the following illustration.

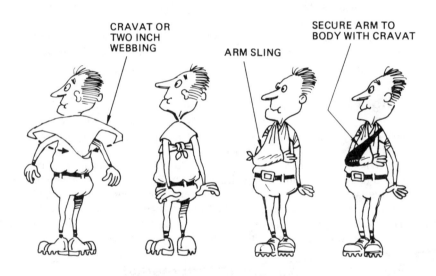

CRAVAT OR TWO INCH WEBBING

ARM SLING

SECURE ARM TO BODY WITH CRAVAT

Lower leg fractures (tibia and fibula)

Again, the basic steps followed for splinting fractures of the forearm should be applied when splinting a lower extremity. The following specifics, however, apply:

  1. Splint by using an ice ax or branch on the outside of the injured leg AND by using the adjacent uninjured leg. A second ice ax between the legs can be used but it is not required.

2. If an ice ax is used, the spike end should be pointing toward the waist and the pick up (adze down). This position allows for least interference with transportation and allows the ankle to be secured to the ice ax head. Be careful to pad both the spike and the pick with tape, a sock, or a hat.

3. Pad between the legs and all splinting material.

4. If straightening of the extremity is required to effectively splint and transport the victim, carefully place it in a normal position by grasping the foot with one hand over the instep and the other hand at the heel and firmly exerting a gentle pull. If resistance is felt or if the victim's pain does not tolerate the move, splint it as is and make special transportation arrangements.

5. Remember elevation. When the splint is complete, elevate the leg 4 to 6 inches, supporting it EVENLY. Do not allow the heel to rest on the ground. Keep the knee slightly flexed.

Fracture of the kneecap (patella)

Immobilize the knee joint by placing a splint underneath the knee extending from the buttock to the heel. It must be well padded under the knee and ankle to keep them in a slightly bent, more natural position. Avoid tying webbing directly over the kneecap but rather above and below.

Fracture of the thigh (femur)

A fracture of the femur is extremely serious and perhaps the most painful of all fractures. The muscles in the thigh area are extremely powerful and there is substantial bone override, sometimes as much as 3 inches. The result is that broken bone ends protrude into the surrounding tissue, causing internal bleeding and sometimes nerve damage. One method to reduce the amount of override is traction splinting. If it is done properly, it is extremely worthwhile if lengthy transportation or transportation over rough terrain is necessary. Methods normally employed involve the use of the half-ring (Keller-Blake) or full-ring (Thomas) splint. The techniques for the use of these splints, however, are involved, must be done well, and take considerable time and manpower to accomplish properly.

In a mountaineering situation, these materials are obviously not available. At best, a splint could be improvised with well padded branches, skis, ski poles, or ice axes. However, other than with ideal equipment in ideal conditions, the disadvantages of traction splinting outweigh the advantages. Some of these disadvantages are:

1. Unless applied extremely well (professionally), restricting cravats will cut off or impede circulation. During the long wait for outside assistance (12 hours or more), tissue damage will almost certainly occur.

2. In order to apply enough traction to relieve pain and control bone overriding, cravats and splinting material must be used properly. It would be disastrous if the splint were to break or a cravat suddenly slip during transportation.

3. Once traction is applied, the leg must be kept elevated.

For these reasons, then, APPLICATION OF A TRACTION SPLINT IN MOUNTAINEERING SITUATIONS IS DISCOURAGED.

In the case of an open fracture, the bone end should not be left exposed. Before straightening the limb, thereby allowing the bone to slip back under the skin, examine the end carefully for dirt and debris. DO NOT HANDLE the bone end. If dirty it should be rinsed with a saline solution of 1 teaspoon of salt, or 12 salt tablets, in a quart of clean, or preferably sterile, water. In all cases NEVER allow the bone to dry out—keep it wet. DO NOT attempt to push the bone under the skin but let it slip back of its own accord when the limb is straightened.

Splint carefully, fully immobilizing above and below the fracture. Keep the injured area accessible so that it can periodically be observed. In the case of an open fracture, place a tourniquet LOOSELY above the fracture for use if bleeding becomes uncontrollable and cannot be stopped by any other means. For a fracture of the femur, the outside splint should be extended alongside the body to a point just below the armpit and held in place at several points by seven or eight ties extending completely around the chest and abdomen. Be sure the blood supply has not been shut off; check frequently for swelling and blueness. Pad between the legs before they are tied together. Secure the arms for evacuation.

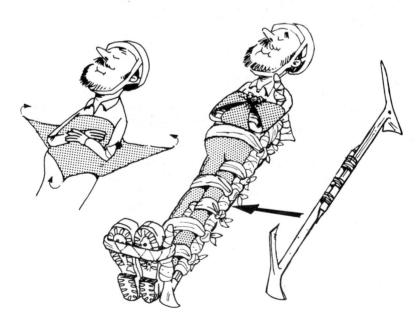

Fracture of the pelvis

Fractures of the pelvis are usually caused by severe trauma and may be accompanied by internal injuries of the digestive, urinary, or genital systems. Blood in the urine, for example, is definitely a sign of bladder damage.

If a pelvic fracture is suspected, with or without internal injury, the victim should be placed on his back with knees flexed. He should not be allowed to stand or walk. If he complains of pain in the hip region when moving a lower extremity, consider a fracture of the neck of the femur (rather than pelvis) and splint from the armpit to the heel with a thick pad between the thighs.

Fracture of the ribs (discussed under chest injuries)

Fracture of the skull

All injuries to the skull are potentially life-threatening. Their seriousness depends upon the degree of damage to the brain rather than exclusively on the physical damage to the skull itself. Generally, if the victim has not lost consciousness, there is reasonable assurance that no major injury exists. If the victim lost consciousness for a brief time (a few minutes) but he responds when his name is called or responds to pinching or other pain stimulus, he most likely has sustained a contusion or mild bruising of the brain. Although there may or may not be external bleeding, his injury would be considered minor if his condition continues to improve with time.

Skull fracture symptoms

Minor Injury or Immediate Symptoms	Major Injury or Later Symptoms
Headache and localized pain	Prolonged unconsciousness
Pulse full and slow	Blood or cerebrospinal fluid from the ears, nose, or mouth
Facial color reddish	Pulse weak and rapid
Minor scalp bleeding	Face color ashen
Bump on head where struck	Breathing labored and heavy
Consciousness	Changes in eye pupils (unequal in size, dilated and not responsive to light)
	Paralysis
	Skull indented or soft where struck

IF, however, the victim:

1. Lost consciousness for a relatively long period of time (20 minutes or more),
2. Was conscious or semiconscious at first but gradually lost consciousness,
3. Regained consciousness but slipped back into an unconscious state, OR
4. Remained conscious but exhibited symptoms of major injury, then SEVERE BRAIN DAMAGE SHOULD BE SUSPECTED; immediate hospitalization and medical care are required.

The first aid administered to the victim of a head injury depends upon the severity of the injury. For minor injuries, for example, in which there is relatively little bleeding from the scalp, the first aid is the same as for any minor wound: bandage. The victim may then be allowed to walk out.

If the victim lost consciousness briefly, however, before being allowed to get up, he should be examined thoroughly to determine what injury has taken place. He should be asked, for example, to add some one digit numbers, or who is the president, etc. to determine if his reasoning and memory are normal. He should be tested for balance, coordination, and vision during a "trial" walk. If no abnormalities appear and if he complains ONLY of minor injury symptoms at most, he may be allowed to walk out WITH ASSISTANCE AND CONSTANT OBSERVATION. It should be

First aid for head injuries

Minor injury		Major injury
Allow to walk with assistance	**Wait for help**	**Evacuate immediately**
Very brief unconsciousness if at all	Unconscious 5 to 20 minutes	Unconsciousness 20 or more minutes
Victim improved and appears normal	Victim does not appear to be improving	Drifts back into unconsciousness
Victim feels he is able to travel	Victim feels sick and nauseous	Exhibits other signs of major head injury
Bleeding controlled	Generalized head throbbing	Vital signs deteriorating
	Route out difficult and long	

noted that even though no signs and symptoms of major injury were observed at the time of the accident, a blood clot may form within the skull or internal bleeding can occur which could prove fatal some time later.

If the victim has lost consciousness for 5 to 20 minutes, complains of feeling sick and nauseous, has a generalized throbbing, and the route out is long and difficult, it is better to wait for assistance rather than risk further harm during evacuation.

Finally, if the victim exhibits signs of MAJOR head injury or worsening condition, he should be EVACUATED IMMEDIATELY. The need for prompt medical attention is urgent. Possible additional injury occurring during the evacuation is of less importance than immediate medical attention WHEN THE VICTIM'S CONDITION IS PROGRESSIVELY DETERIORATING. CAUTION: ALWAYS suspect a neck injury. Approximately 15% of all severe head injuries are associated with a broken neck.

Fracture of the spine

Whenever a person has a pain in the neck or back following an accident, always consider the possibility of spinal fracture even though local swelling and tenderness are absent.

Fractures of the neck (cervical vertebrae) are most frequently caused by a blow on the head during a fall or by a falling rock. Examination for neck injury should always be conducted simultaneously with examination for a head injury.

1. Determine if the victim's neck hurts. If pain is severe, even if there are no local bruises, suspect a neck fracture or hemorrhage in the membranes covering the spinal cord.
2. Do not ask the victim to move his head. With a broken neck he is apt to have a great deal of muscular spasm and will not want to do so.
3. If other injuries permit, test for:
   a. Loss of muscular power in the arms or legs by asking the victim to move them carefully against some resistance.
   b. Loss of sensation. Pinch various parts of the victim's body asking if sensation is felt. Always check both right and left sides. Paralysis of the upper extremities indicates probable cervical injury.
4. If doubt remains concerning the presence of a neck fracture, treat the victim as though he had one.

Before performing first aid, it must be realized that any forward or backward flexation may sever the spinal cord, causing permanent paralysis or death. Therefore, extreme caution must be exercised when splinting or moving the victim.

It is essential that splinting be accomplished prior to moving. There are two splinting methods that can be used. The first and probably the most common, is the use of a neck collar. A padded wire splint approximately 3 to 4 inches wide and 12 inches long, or a padded hip belt from a pack, serve this function well. Either is placed under the chin and around the neck with the two ends joining in the back. This keeps the head supported and prevents movement. CAUTION: use well-padded stiff or rigid materials such as wire or Ensolite only. If the material is loose or unpacked, such as clothing, the head will not be supported rigidly enough to prevent forward flexation. The second method is to place a pad (stuff sack full of clothing, parka, Ensolite, etc.) at the small of the neck. A sling, cravat, or tape is then placed around the forehead, running down the back, crossing and under the armpits around the chest. This will keep the head, neck, and chest in a straight line and even slightly arched backwards. Before performing either method, properly size the splint and practice the technique on an uninjured member of the party.

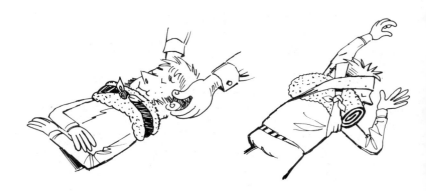

When moving the victim is required to insert insulative materials under him, splint first and then use a "log roll" whereby the victim is turned as a unit with the head and body in perfect alignment. One first aider holds the head in slight traction, rotating it as three assistants simultaneously rotate the trunk and legs. All first aiders kneel with the assistants rotating the victim toward them—NOT away. For easier rolling, the victim's arm on the side on which he will be rolled should be extended above his head out of the way. While the victim is held on his side, insulative materials are then placed beneath him as close as possible and slightly bunched or folded next to him. On command, he is then gently rotated back and the padding carefully straightened to center it. Any other movement prior to transportation is unwise. DO NOT, for example, insert him through the door of a tent. Instead, cut the bottom out of the tent and erect it around him.

For evacuation, the victim must be transported by rigid stretcher. Use of an improvised stretcher is NOT RECOMMENDED. The head must be secured to prevent any movement. This can be done by placing pads on all sides of the head and tying it down with webbing. It should be emphasized that it is just as important to prevent the rest of the body from moving as it is the head. Use of adequate padding keeps the victim from moving and reduces the risk of circulatory impediment from tight webbing or straps.

Fractures of the back (thoracic or lumbar vertebrae) are extremely serious in that displacement or fracturing of the vertebrae can cause puncturing or severing of the spinal cord. If this occurs, it will result in partial or complete paralysis to all areas below the injury. If a person falls and lands on his feet or buttocks, the last two thoracic or any of the lumbar vertebrae are particularly susceptible to being injured. In such an accident:

1. Check for loss of motor power and sensation by asking the injured to move his legs, feet and toes, and by testing his sensitivity to touch. Paralysis of the lower extremities indicates probable thoracic or lumbar spine injury.

2. Determine the location of pain. If it is 2 or 3 inches to one side of the midline, there is probably a fracture of a transverse process (bony projection on either side of a vertebra). Pain which is deeper and in the midline of the spine indicates fractures of the vertebral body (main weight-bearing structure of the vertebra).

There is little that can be done from a first aid standpoint. If ground insulation is needed, log roll the victim, keeping his legs constantly in line with his body. Place insulative materials underneath him including a small pad under the back to hyperextend it. With hyperextension, there is less likelihood of further injury to the spinal cord. If there is any doubt regarding a possible back injury, send for help so that evacuation can be accomplished by rigid stretcher.

injuries to joints and muscles

Sprains

Sprains are torn or stretched soft tissue surrounding joints—ligaments, muscle tendons, blood vessels. Such injury usually causes local hemorrhaging and results in painful swelling.

First aid involves, first, stopping the hemorrhaging by elevation and immediate application of cold compresses locally at the affected joints. Compresses should continue to be applied for at least one hour. They should not be applied, however, if the victim is suffering from general cooling; it is more important to keep him warm. Taping an ankle or the application of a figure-eight ankle bandage provides some relief from pain. Generally, however, unless the first aider is skilled in applying tape and has been trained how to do so, taping is best left to a physician. If pain persists and there is doubt as to a sprain or a fracture, play it safe: SPLINT IT AS IF IT WERE A FRACTURE. No harm is done and, perhaps, much pain and permanent injury will be prevented.

Strains

Strains are overextended or torn muscular fiber. Usually there is little hemorrhaging and usually the injury is not associated with a joint. In these cases, warm compresses should be applied to aid circulation and promote healing.

Dislocations

Dislocations are often obviously evidenced by visual deformity and severe pain. Correction of a dislocation is technically difficult, and unskilled efforts can damage blood vessels and nerves, or even produce fractures. Such injuries should be regarded as fractures and NO ATTEMPT AT RELOCATION MADE. An exception might be the relocation of a finger, which may be attempted only if medical help is distant and pain severe.

chest
injuries

There are two probable types of injuries to the chest that can occur in a mountaineering situation: falling on an ice ax or sharp branch in such a way that there is a penetration into the chest cavity and perhaps a puncture of the lungs; and falling while roped with a bowline such that the coil slips over the ribs, fracturing them. These two cases will be discussed separately.

Rib fractures

Ribs may be fractured with the bone ends remaining in place, with the ends projecting outward, or with the ends projecting inward. In any case most often there is little or no noticeable swelling or deformity. Breathing causes pain, which is usually quite localized, and detectable by running the fingers along the ribs or by compression of the rib cage. NOTE: when checking for tenderness and isolating the area of the fracture, do not do so through a parka. Get down to a thin shirt or bare skin.

The first aid for fractured ribs depends upon the position of the broken ends. If they are in place or outward, the objective for treating fractures is followed (splint). In this case, splinting is best done by securing at least three cravats or three strips of webbing around the chest cavity, restricting movements of the fractured bones. This not only keeps the broken bones quiet but reduces pain associated with their movement. A more secure splint can be improvised by placing a forearm diagonally across the area, and binding it in place also. This, too, aids in reducing movement. Binding of the chest should be done as the victim exhales rather than as he inhales.

If the ribs are fractured inward, this may be detected by feeling a cavity or indentation in the area of tenderness. If this is suspected or if compression increases pain, the chest SHOULD NOT be bound, since it may cause the fractured ends to penetrate the pleural cavity or the lungs themselves, causing irreversible damage and possible death. In this case, DO NOT allow the victim to travel under his own power. He must be evacuated.

Puncture wounds of the chest

If the chest has been punctured but the wound appears to be minor (surface penetration only, little bleeding and no difficulty in breathing), treat like any other open wound. Bandage and dress. If, however, penetration is deep, the object may have entered the pleural cavity, causing collapse of a lung. In this case, the wound will admit air from the outside upon inhalation. This can be heard and seen. It is referred to as a "sucking chest wound" or pneumothorax and is, obviously, extremely serious. The first aid should be IMMEDIATE. Apply a plastic bag or piece of thin plastic over the wound to form a positive air-tight seal, thereby excluding any air exchange. (If the victim experiences difficulty in breathing after the seal is applied, it may be lifted briefly to allow trapped air to escape and immediately reapplied.) Place a large pad over the area and bind it in place. The pad assists in maintaining sufficient and uniform pressure on the seal. Laying the victim on his injured side applies additional pressure, ensures a more effective seal, and allows the injured side to work more effectively. Transport the victim in that position (injured side down).

injuries
to the eye

Snowblindness

The surface of the eye, just as the skin, is sensitive to ultraviolet radiation. The higher the altitude, the greater the exposure to ultraviolet. If exposure is extensive, a burn of its surface and surrounding tissues will occur resulting in what is known as snowblindness. Its symptoms, like those of a sunburn, usually do not become apparent for many hours, sometimes eight to twelve, after exposure. The eyes feel irritated and dry at first but later feel as if they are "full of sand." Moving and blinking is extremely painful and tearing profuse. The eyelids are often red and swollen, and difficult if not impossible to keep open.

Obviously better than first aid is prevention. Individuals traveling on snow for more than an hour or two should wear dark goggles or sunglasses with side shields. Lenses should not transmit more than 20% of the visible light and essentially none below 3600A in the ultraviolet. CAUTION: many sunglasses sold for driving do NOT provide adequate protection for prolonged use on snow. Accept the need to carry spare goggles or lenses. In an emergency situation, a lens of cardboard or other suitable material with a slit cut horizontally or pinholes at each eye position can be improvised. An alternate approach is to tape a strip of "Space Blanket" over the eyes (reflecting side outward).

Snowblindness will heal in a few days. Cold compresses and eye bandages will give some relief, but various ointments in the eye can be damaging and should not be used, except as prescribed by a physician. The victim should be cautioned against rubbing the eyes and perhaps causing an infection. Evacuation by stretcher may be required in severe cases.

Objects in the eye

Getting "something in the eye" in the mountains is common since winds and people above you are also common. In most instances, natural watering is sufficient to dislodge and wash away any object. Occasionally, however, perhaps as a result of a fall, objects become lodged and cannot easily be removed. What to do depends upon the severity of the injury. In the case where a foreign body lodges on the surface of the eye, immediate irrigation with water may dislodge it. The fluid should be poured into the inner corner of the eye and allowed to run over the eyeball while the lid is gently lifted by the lashes. Obviously the eye should not be rubbed. If irrigation fails, and the object can be seen, the first aider may try to gently lift it with a moist corner of a sterile guaze pad.

If the object is protruding from the eye, the situation clearly is much more serious. The first aid for such injuries is as follows:

1. No attempt to remove the object or to wash the eye should be made. Leave the object alone.
2. Using a cravat or clothing, improvise a donut to encircle the protruding object.

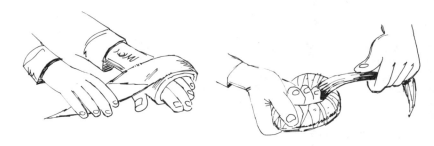

3. Bandage over both eyes, being careful not to disturb the protruding object. The rule is to "protect from further harm."
4. Carry the victim on his back by stretcher to medical aid. Do not allow him to walk or use the other eye, since sympathetic eye movement can result in more harm and definitely more pain.

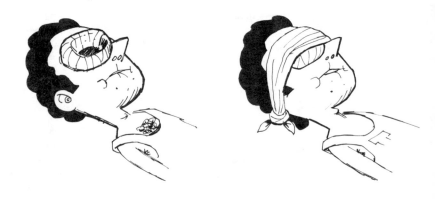

Contact lenses

Although contact lenses in themselves are safe, they can be harmful to an unconscious individual if left unattended. Consequently, it is important for the first aider to determine if the victim is wearing contacts and respond appropriately.

First, to determine if the victim has contact lenses in place, raise the eyelids and look from the side at the cornea. In almost all cases the lenses will be readily visible. If, upon searching through the victim's belongings, a contact lens case or wetting solution are found, this, too, will provide a good clue that the victim is wearing contacts.

Second, determine the type of lens. The most popular are the corneal lenses slightly less in diameter than the colored part of the eye. If they are being worn, rather than removing them, simply slide each lens, with clean hands, to the white part of the eye. There they will be safe until the victim can be transported to professional help. If the lenses are the larger soft type, covering all of the colored part of the eye and some of the white, proceed as follows: with clean hands, place one finger to the outside edge of the lower eyelid. Carefully open the lid until the edge of the lens becomes visible. While maintaining pressure, slide the finger toward the victim's ear, pulling the eyelid taut. This should cause the lid to slide under the lens, lifting the edge so that it can be grasped for removal. When removed, place the lens in the victim's container or some other hard container with clean water.

effects
of excessive
heat

The body reacts to increase in temperature in two ways: by dilating the surface blood vessels, thereby allowing more body-warmed blood to pass near the skin surface to be cooled through the skin by conduction, convection, and radiation; and by perspiring, thereby causing cooling by evaporation. When heat cannot be lost by the body fast enough to keep it cool, the body's temperature will rise, resulting in a burn, heat exhaustion, heat stroke, or heat cramps.

Burns

Burns are classified according to severity or degree:

1st degree — A reddening of the skin, such as sunburn.

2nd degree — A deeper burn with blistering.

3rd degree — A burn causing underlying tissue damage, charring and cell destruction.

The general objective when performing first aid is to relieve pain by excluding air, preventing contamination and treating for shock. Since the manner in which this is done varies with burn severity, some estimate of the severity must be made before performing first aid.

Prevention of **sunburn** is obviously more effective than any first aid that can be administered. For the first outing of the season on snow, for example, an exposure of more than 15 minutes without protection should be avoided. Later in the season, after tanning, the exposure time may be lengthened, although almost never to the point of not requiring a protective cream for continuous glacier travel. Lightweight hats, scarves, or handkerchiefs worn about the head also provide protection from sunburn. Regardless of how bizarre the effect, the use of hats and scarves is extremely worthwhile. Additionally, one may use protective creams or ointments. For maximum protection frequent application of creams and ointments such as zinc oxide, A-Fil, Sun Guard or U-Val is required. For less protection, creams such as Neo-A-Fil or "Snootie" may be used. For minimum protection Sea and Ski, Copper Tone, etc., are available. The effectiveness of these varies dramatically from individual to individual. For glacier travel, one should choose a preparation which provides good protection and ideally:

1. Will not dissolve in perspiration or rub off easily.
2. Is easily removed with soap and water.
3. Blocks ultraviolet radiation.

It should be noted that some individuals may be allergic to brands mentioned above and/or others.

If preventive measures have not been taken and a sunburn has been incurred, the first aid is the application of a salt-free lotion (sometimes referred to as a burn lotion). Its main function is to exclude air. Little else can be done.

For **second degree burns** the application of a lotion to relieve pain is NOT recommended. Rather, the body part should be immediately immersed in cold water or covered with snow for up to 30 minutes or until the pain has subsided. If the part cannot be immersed in water or covered with snow, cloths wrung out in cold water should be applied. Blot the area dry and cover with at least six layers of dry sterile dressing.

For **third degree burns** the application of a lotion and/or the immersion of the injured part in cold water are NOT recommended. These not only cause possible contamination of the wound, but in the case of immersion, further physical damage. It is best to cover with sterile dressings to prevent contamination, and to wrap the area in plastic to exclude air and keep the underlying dressings clean. Ice packs can then be applied on top of the plastic to relieve pain. Position the victim and administer fluids as in the first aid treatment for shock.

Heat exhaustion

Heat exhaustion may occur either when an individual is exposed to a hot environment or when the individual, because of physical exertion, overheats. The surrounding air temperature may or may not be high. In heat exhaustion, the blood vessels in the skin become so dilated that blood to the brain and other vital organs is reduced to inadequate levels. The resultant physiological condition is similar to fainting. The victim usually feels nauseous, restless, dizzy, thirsty, and may have a headache. His temperature, however, is not significantly elevated and, in fact, may be below normal. Sweating is generally profuse and the skin color is pale. An individual is significantly more susceptible to heat exhaustion with even minor degrees of dehydration or salt deficiency.

The first aid for heat exhaustion is to lay the victim in a cool, shady environment. Administer a salt solution of approximately 1 teaspoon (12 tablets) of salt in a quart of water. Recovery will usually be very rapid.

Heat stroke

Heat stroke (sometimes called "sunstroke") results from an inadequacy of the sweating process. For normal individuals exercising in a hot environment, the rate of sweating decreases steadily. After a number of hours of uninterrupted work the rate of perspiration usually reaches very low levels but is still adequate to cool the body. In heat stroke, the sweating process and other body heat regulatory mechanisms have failed. (This sweating deficiency appears to result from exhaustion of the sweat glands.) Consequently, the individual's temperature rises. HEAT STROKE IS EXTREMELY DANGEROUS!

The onset of heat stroke is often very rapid. The victim may be previously aware of extreme heat, but then quickly becomes confused, uncoordinated, delirious, or unconscious. Characteristically, the body temperature is above 105° F, the skin is hot, red in color, and sweating is absent. The condition is frequently observed in the aged, alcoholics, or obese persons but is by no means confined to them.

It is important to decrease body temperature IMMEDIATELY by cold water applications. Remove or unfasten clothing. Shade the body. Reduce the victim's temperature to approximately 103° or lower.

Heat cramps

Muscular cramps (usually abdominal or in the limbs) are caused by lactic acid accumulating in muscular tissues, and as a result of salt deficiency through prolonged perspiration. The condition can occur either because of a shortage of salt or water, or both combined with physical exercise.

The first step in treatment is to allow the victim to lie down and rest, thereby allowing the blood to carry away lactic acid accumulations. Firmly support the cramped muscle and stretch it. Administer a salt solution to remove the underlying cause. Avoid further strenuous exercise, if possible, until fully rested and rehydrated.

effects
of excessive
cold

Frostbite

One way in which the body protects itself during cold weather is to constrict surface blood vessels (other than those of the head and neck). This mechanism reduces the blood flowing to the body surfaces, thereby holding a larger percentage of the total supply in the body's inner core and allowing vital body functions to be maintained at a constant temperature. The hands have the greatest skin area for their volume of any part of the body and therefore cool very rapidly. Additionally, since the hands and feet are also the farthest away from the heart, the flow of blood to those extremities is poorest and surface blood vessel constriction affects them the most. (Remember the saying "Cold hands, warm heart"?) The ears and nose, although receiving a great amount of blood, protrude from the body and are, therefore, quite susceptible to cooling.

Primarily, then, when the body requires increased central blood flow to assure warmth of the core and brain, the surface blood vessels are contracted and the skin cools. If cooling is continued, underlying muscles are affected and coordination becomes more difficult. It becomes more difficult to strike a match, tie a cord, or handle a small object. As the skin temperature drops below 50°F, all sense of touch and pain are lost. If the temperature continues to drop, circulation will almost completely cease and "frostbite" will occur. The water in the cells between the skin and capillaries freezes. Tissues are injured physically from the expansion of the ice and by the resultant chemical imbalance within each cell.

Frostbite can be prevented. One should not be exposed to the cold when exhausted or not well. Accept the need to wear enough clothing, including an outer garment of plastic or coated nylon to protect against the wind, an extra pair of woolen socks, mittens rather than gloves, and head protection. If a part becomes cold, place it against a warm body part or cover it more. Some physical activity, especially exercising of the fingers and toes, is helpful. Avoid alcoholic drinks and smoking immediately before and during exposure. (Smoking constricts surface blood vessels in the extremities, thus increasing the likelihood of frostbite.) Do not touch supercooled metal or liquids with bare hands or lips.

The symptoms of frostbite, like those of a burn, vary in degree of severity and extent. Regrettably, in many instances, not until many days after exposure has occurred, can the extent or severity be accurately determined. For this reason, frostbite is divided into two general categories — superficial and deep.

In cases of superficial frostbite, the skin appears pale, grayish-white in color. This can be observed at normal room temperature by pushing with a finger against another body part temporarily impeding circulation to that area. When removing the finger, the area will momentarily appear grayish-white until the blood returns. In superficial frostbite, too, the skin is hard and appears frozen although the deeper tissues remain soft and resilient. Pain is usually felt early but later subsides. The part feels intensely cold or numb.

In cases of deep frostbite, not only is the superficial surface tissue hard, but the underlying tissue, as well, is hard and solid. Freezing will extend to the muscles and even the bone itself. The area has no feeling — pain is absent.

Immediate **first aid for superficial frostbite** is to cover the frozen part with dry, insulating, windproof material, and place a warm body part next to it, applying firm, steady pressure. DO NOT RUB the area with a hand or in the snow. Experience has shown that rubbing the injured tissue increases the risk of tissue death (gangrene). Get the victim indoors or into a tent where more complete first aid can be given. Once the victim is inside a shelter, proper thawing is best accomplished by rapidly immersing the part in water slightly warmer than body temperature (102°F to 105°F). At least one 1½-ounce, −40°F to 120°F, thermometer should be carried by every party. Do not apply hot water bottles or heat lamps, or place the frozen part near a hot stove, because excessive heat may increase the damage. If water is not available, rewarm with another body part. If the toes are frostbitten, for example, apply the old mountaineering remedy — a bare foot against a climbing companion's bare stomach. Give the victim warm food and drink (non-alcoholic), and encourage him to exercise injured fingers and toes. Do not disturb blisters, should they appear, since the possibility of infection is great. Maintain the most sterile conditions possible.

First aid for deep frostbite is quite another matter. If the signs of deep frostbite are evident, if deep frostbite is suspected, or if it is impossible to get an individual into shelter where complete and uninterrupted thawing can be accomplished, thawing SHOULD NOT be attempted. Once thawing of a deeply frostbitten or frozen extremity is begun, the victim will immediately become a litter case. Therefore, if it is necessary for him to assist in his rescue, thawing is best delayed. Evidence indicates that a delay of up to 24 hours makes relatively little difference in the ultimate outcome. Under no conditions should a thawed or partially thawed part be allowed to refreeze. This invariably causes far greater and more serious tissue destruction. When and if the victim is properly sheltered, thaw the affected part by immersion as with superficial frostbite. Warm, body-temperature water (90°F to 104°F) is best. Complete, uninterrupted thawing under STERILE conditions is a requirement.

Exposure

Exposure, referring to the medical condition, is more accurately defined as a combination of factors leading to physiological deterioration, and frequently to death. Deaths from exposure, in the United States, amount to about 10 per cent of the total mountaineering mishaps. The important factors of exposure are hypothermia (a lowering of the temperature of the body's inner core), inadequate food consumption, dehydration, and overexertion.

Although not all factors may be present, any one or combination of these may cause death from exposure. For example, an individual climbing for a long time in cold weather may become exhausted. Additionally, he may not have consumed a sufficient amount of food and drink. As a result, moving very slowly, he will not be capable of generating enough heat to maintain a constant body temperature. Without sufficient food, heat cannot be generated through food oxidation. Therefore, heat loss exceeds heat gain and the individual collapses, losing consciousness and, unless the situation is corrected, dies. This condition, it should be noted, can occur at temperatures well above freezing when precipitated by the factors listed above.

Each of these factors will be discussed in detail: inadequate food consumption, dehydration, and overexertion are described later under Effects of Extreme and Prolonged Exertion.

Hypothermia

To understand hypothermia it is useful to review some basic concepts of how the body can gain and lose heat. The body gains or conserves heat in four ways:

1. Through the digestion of food. The body produces heat by oxidation of food and tissue at a specific rate while resting (called the basal metabolic rate) or at an increased rate while exercising.

2. Externally. Examples are hot food and drink, sun, fire, another body, etc.

3. Through muscular activity, either by deliberate exercise or by involuntary exercise like shivering. Shivering produces as much heat as running at a slow pace or the approximate equivalent to the amount of heat generated from eating two medium size chocolate bars per hour.

4. Through constriction of surface blood vessels. Constriction of surface blood vessels reduces circulation at the skin layers and blood is kept nearer to the central core of the body.

The body loses heat in five ways:

1. Respiration. A large amount of heat escapes when we exhale warm air. This cannot be prevented entirely (unless we stop breathing) but it can be reduced. This is accomplished by covering the mouth/nose area with wool or other insulative material, thereby "pre-warming" the air as it passes through the material.

2. Evaporation. As discussed under Heat Exhaustion, evaporation of perspiration from the skin and lungs contributes greatly to the amount of heat lost by the body. One-twentieth of a fluid ounce of perspiration evaporates and cools the body approximately 2°F. Although this cannot be prevented, the amount of evaporation (and therefore cooling) can be controlled by wearing clothing that can be opened easily for ventilation or taken off readily, and by wearing clothing that won't absorb water but will breathe, i.e., let the water vapor escape.

3. Conduction. Sitting on the snow, touching cold equipment, being rained upon, etc., are all examples of how heat can be lost as a result of conduction. As mentioned earlier, if an individual becomes wet, a tremendous amount of body heat is lost rapidly. Deaths have occurred as a result of invididuals being suspended in or immersed in water below 40°F in which the body temperature could not be maintained. Although not as immediately serious in mountaineering situations, try never to allow perspiration to saturate articles of clothing. Their insulative properties are obviously seriously reduced.

4. Radiation. This causes the greatest amount of heat loss from the body from uncovered surfaces, particularly the head, neck, and hands. Coverage of these areas, therefore, is extremely important in keeping warm.

5. Convection. The body continually warms (by radiation) a thin layer of air next to the skin. If warm air is retained close to the body, it remains warm. If removed by wind or air currents (convection), it cools. The primary function of clothing is to retain this layer of warm air next to the skin while allowing water vapor to pass outward. It does this by enclosing air in cell walls or between numerous fibers. Heat is lost rapidly with the lightest breeze unless the proper type of clothing is worn to prevent the warm air from being convected away.

Deaths have been attributed to a loss of body heat at temperatures of 40°F, with 30 mph breeze. Under these conditions, the cooling effect on the skin is equal to that of much lower temperatures due to increased evaporation and convection. At lower temperatures and strong winds, cooling occurs even more rapidly. This is why the victim of an accident situation must have wind protection to ensure that his body heat will not be carried away. This is why he must also be provided with a great deal of insulation (dead air space) to ensure that body heat is retained at safe levels.

If heat loss exceeds heat gain, and if the condition is allowed to continue, hypothermia results. The first response to exposure to cold is constriction of the blood vessels of the skin and, later, of the deeper lying tissue. The effect is to decrease the amount of heat transported by blood to the skin, consequently lowering skin temperature. The cool shell of skin now acts as an insulating layer for the deeper core areas of the body; skin temperatures may drop nearly as low as that of the surrounding environment, while the body's core temperature remains unchanged at its normal 98.6 degrees. However, a drop to 50° F, always numbs the skin so that ultimately all sense of touch and pain is lost, rendering the hands, for example, almost useless in performing fine or coordinated movement. Shivering begins shortly after the initial constriction of surface blood vessels and may continue for several hours if exposure to cold is continued. Although it produces considerable heat, shivering consumes a great deal of energy, and if intense and prolonged can result in exhaustion. Inevitably, if this heat loss continues, the body's inner core temperature begins to fall below 98.6 degrees. As this occurs, body functions are impaired, the victim loses coordination and eventually consciousness. If the situation is not quickly remedied, he dies.

The insidious nature of hypothermia is its absence of warning to the victim, and the fact that as its severity increases, chilling reaches his brain, thus depriving him of the judgment and reasoning power to recognize his own condition. Without recognition of symptoms by a companion, and treatment, this vicious cycle leads to stupor, collapse, and death.

The following table presents a summary of signs and symptoms keyed to the body's inner core (rectal) temperature. The temperatures shown are only approximate, nor can they be measured in the field since normal medical thermometers read only as low as 94°F. However, the table provides an indication of how the bodily functions deteriorate with falling core temperatures. Learn to recognize these signs and symptoms and carefully watch yourself as well as others in your party during exposure to cold, wet, and wind.

There are four lines of defense against hypothermia:

1. **Avoidance of exposure.** In avoiding exposure dress for warmth, wind, and wet. When clothes become wet, they lose about 90 per cent of their insulating value. Wind drives cold air under and through clothing and refrigerates wet clothing by evaporating moisture from the surface. Put on rain gear before becoming wet; put on wool clothes and wind gear before shivering starts. Do not be deceived by temperatures well above freezing; most hypothermia cases develop in air temperatures between 30°F and 50°F, and water at 50°F is unbearably cold, particularly when it is running down the neck and legs and flushing body heat from the surface of

Effects of Hypothermia

TREATMENT

Reduce Heat Loss

Add Heat

SIGNS AND SYMPTOMS

Body Inner Core Symptoms	Observable in Others	Felt by Yourself
Intense and uncontrollable shivering; ability to perform complex tasks impaired.	Slowing of pace Intense shivering Poor coordination	Fatigue. Uncontrollable fits of shivering. Immobile, fumbling hands.
Violent shivering persists, difficulty in speaking, sluggish thinking, amnesia begins to appear.	Stumbling, lurching gait. Thickness of speech. Poor judgment.	Stumbling. Poor articulation. Feeling of deep cold or numbness.
Shivering decreases; replaced by muscular rigidity and erratic, jerky movements; thinking not clear but maintains posture.	Irrationality, incoherence. Amnesia, memory lapses. Hallucinations. Loss of contact with environment.	Disorientation. Decrease in shivering. Stiffening of muscles. Exhaustion, inability to get up after a rest.
Victim becomes irrational, loses contact with environment, drifts into stupor; muscular rigidity continues; pulse and respiration slowed.	Blueness of skin. Decreased heart and respiratory rate. Dilation of pupils. Weak or irregular pulse. Stupor.	Blueness of skin. Slow, irregular, or weak pulse. Drowsiness.
Unconsciousness; does not respond to spoken word; most reflexes cease to function; heartbeat becomes erratic.	Unconsciousness	
Failure of cardiac and respiratory control centers in brain; cardiac fibrillation; probable edema and hemorrhage in lungs. Death.		

the clothes. The question is not how cold is the air, but instead, how cold is the water against the body.

2. **Termination of exposure.** If you cannot stay dry and warm under the existing conditions, terminate exposure by getting out of the wind and rain. Bivouac early before energy is exhausted and before coordination and judgment are impaired. Eat sweets which are quickly and easily absorbed and keep continuously active to ensure adequate heat production.

3. **Early detection.** Any time a party is exposed to wind, cold, or wet, carefully watch each individual for the symptoms of hypothermia: uncontrollable fits of shivering; vague, slow, slurred speech; irrational actions; memory lapses, incoherence; immobile, fumbling hands; frequent stumbling, lurching gait; apparent exhaustion, inability to get up after a rest; drowsiness (to sleep is to die). Below the critical body heat temperature of 95°F the victim cannot produce enough body heat by himself to recover. At this point extreme measures must be taken to reverse the dropping core temperature. Remember that a person may slip into hypother-

60

mia in a matter of minutes and can die in less than 2 hours after the first signs of hypothermia are detected.

4. **Immediate treatment.** Although the victim may deny he is in trouble, BELIEVE THE SYMPTOMS, NOT THE VICTIM. Even mild symptoms demand immediate, drastic treatment. First, prevent any further heat loss by getting the victim out of the wind and rain and into the best shelter available. Then remove his wet clothing and replace it with dry garments, insulate him from the ground, and warm him by the most expedient methods available. If the victim is only mildly impaired give him warm drinks and get him into a sleeping bag prewarmed by another member of the party who has stripped to his underclothing in order to transfer a maximum amount of heat from his body to the bag. (Placing a hypothermia victim in a cold sleeping bag, no matter how much down it contains, is not sufficient because the victim's body cannot produce the heat needed to warm the bag and himself.) Well-wrapped, warm (not hot) rocks or canteens also help. Skin-to-skin contact is the most effective treatment, the stripped victim in a sleeping bag with another person (also stripped) or if a double bag is available, between two warmth donors. Build a fire, if possible, on each side of the victim. If he is able to eat he should be fed candy or sweetened foods; carbohydrates are the fuel most quickly transformed into heat and energy. If the victim is semiconscious or worse, try to keep him awake and give him warm drinks (tea, broth, sweetened juice).

effects of extreme and prolonged exertion

Anyone frequenting the outdoors will sooner or later encounter someone suffering from excessive physical fatigue, dehydration, and/or apparent lack of motivation to continue. This is particularly true in hard climbing or backpacking situations where individuals either don't have time or don't take time for a number of physiological necessities — eating, drinking, and rest. Most often the first indication will be that the individual will slow down, gasp for air, complain of being very weak, dizzy, nauseated, or have a headache. All of these symptoms may exist simultaneously or perhaps only one or two will be evidenced. The first aider should ask the following questions:

1. What have you had to eat today? (Remember, two eggs for breakfast doesn't count; it's quickly digested carboyhdrates like candy that are important.)
2. How much liquid have you consumed? (It doesn't matter if it's cold and overcast; if the individual has been working hard, he needs water. If he hasn't consumed at least a quart, his water balance is probably inadequate.)
3. Have you had any salt?
4. Have you done this sort of thing before this year? i.e., are you in condition?

More than likely the victim's answer will be no to at least one question — perhaps to all. In this case, it is best to sit him down and administer a warm, salted, sugar solution. If this is done promptly there is a 90 per cent chance that in 15 minutes the individual will feel tremendously improved and will want to continue (assuming he was properly motivated to begin). Let us examine why this is so.

Inadequate food consumption

An average adult requires approximately 5000 calories per day for heavy activity. This is equivalent to eating 250 packs of Life Savers, 70 cookies, or four loaves of bread per day — an enormous amount of energy. To accomplish this, or at least its equivalent, a conscientious intake of food should be maintained in small quantities every 2 to 4 hours. Diets should contain large quantities of carbohydrates which are quickly converted into glucose and carried into the blood stream. They should not, however, be to the exclusion of fatty foods and proteins. Even though fats and proteins take considerably longer to digest, it is important that they be consumed at regular intervals, thus providing long-range body-building energy. "Gorp," a mixture of candy, raisins, nuts, etc., is both a popular and effective food for providing the body with quick and long-lasting energy.

Dehydration and salt deficiency

As the body exerts itself and heat builds, it perspires. During strenuous activity, particularly at high altitude, the amount of fluids lost through perspiration and evaporation of moisture from the lungs may be as much as five quarts or more per day. If a substantial amount of fluid is lost and not replaced, the body's chemical equilibrium is upset, which may interfere with normal circulation. As this occurs, the symptoms of dehydration and loss of body salts appear. They include: headache, unusual tiredness, weakness, dizziness, nausea, muscular cramps, thirst, dry or sore throat, and, most importantly, an increased tendency to develop severe shock following even a minor injury.

It may be noted that these signs of dehydration and the physiological effects on the body are the same as for heat exhaustion. The only difference is that the victim may feel cold in a cold environment. Nonetheless, a chemical imbalance still exists and must be corrected. As a general guide to prevention and first aid:

1. Fluid intake for a 12-hour day of moderate activity should be at least 2 quarts.
2. Fluid intake for a longer climbing day or for more severe activity should be from 2 to 5 quarts, depending upon the altitude, previous day's activities, the climb severity, and the individual himself.
3. If severe dehydration is already evident, 5 or more quarts given at the rate of 1 to 2 cups per hour should be consumed.

In practice, most individuals seldom carry more than a quart of water with them. This, obviously, causes a problem in maintaining adequate fluids. If the party does not have time to stop and melt snow and does not pass streams, then eating snow or ice becomes necessary. This causes no harm other than the general body cooling as these substances are melted and warmed to body temperature in the mouth and stomach. Additional fluid can be obtained by replacing the water with snow as it is consumed from the container. Then, if the air temperature is above 32°F, melting will add to the liquid contents.

If the outing is longer than a day, the evening should be spent consuming enough fluids to reduce any deficiencies; otherwise more severe dehydration occurs the next day. The body cannot continue without adequate fluids, as it can without food, for more than a few days.

In addition to fluids, the body needs salt to replace that lost through perspiration. The average daily requirement is approximately 1 gram, but during periods of heavy exertion can be as much as 5 grams or more per day. These amounts also vary greatly, depending upon individual needs. Most popularly sold salt tablets are 500 milligrams, which means a daily requirement of approximately two tablets. This is, of course, excluding the salt normally obtained from foods or added to foods. Products like beef jerky and sausage, for example, are high in salt content. Generally taking one salt tablet prior to and one during a moderate day's climb is sufficient. As mentioned above, however, individual needs vary greatly and some will require much more salt, possibly eight to ten tablets OR MORE for a long hard day of climbing.

It is important to note that during a strenuous outing, particularly at high altitudes, appetites for food and fluids are generally poor. As a result, much of the physical fatigue and weakness experienced at high altitudes is undoubtedly due to inadequate food consumption and dehydration. A conscientious effort to consume an adequate level of both food and liquid is required.

Overexertion

Extreme and prolonged physical exertion to the point of exhaustion can render an individual a significant burden to any party. Not only will the individual be physically exhausted (i.e., a general muscular fatigue and weakness), but normally mentally exhausted as well. He will often have no concern about what happens to himself or to the other members of the party. Accompanying his general fatigue are usually dehydration, salt depletion and inadequate food consumption, further complicating possible rapid recovery. The party oftentimes will have no choice but to stop and provide aid to the exhausted victim. If they do not, and if an individual in such a state is injured, shock will occur more readily and is much more serious than in a fresh or rested climber. The exhausted individual is much more susceptible to hypothermia and cold injury. Frostbite, for example, occurs more frequently and is more severe than in a well-fed, rested climber.

How does one prevent overexertion? The most obvious answer is to STAY IN SHAPE. Many books have been written about physical conditioning and physical exertion. No attempt will be made here to expand upon these except to provide ONE VERY MINIMAL set of standards: if, for example, an individual hikes or backpacks leisurely on the weekends only, he should run approximately ½ mile three times during the week. If he goes on one-day climbs on the weekends, he should run approximately 1 mile three times a week, and if he goes on full two-day weekend climbs, he should run 2 miles or more three times a week. This accomplishes a number of things:

1. The first exercise period dramatically illustrates the need for more.
2. The outing itself is made more enjoyable.
3. The individual has some reserve for emergencies.
4. Monday morning aches and pains are significantly reduced.

high altitude effects

Mountain sickness

When an individual ascends to altitude rapidly, his body cannot immediately compensate for the reduced amount of oxygen in the atmosphere. The resultant physiological reaction is known as mountain sickness. It can occur as low as 8,000 feet in some individuals and in almost everyone to some extent who ascends higher than 12,000 feet in less than 48 hours.

The symptoms are primarily caused by a lack of sufficient oxygen in the blood and its effect on the brain. They include: nausea, vomiting, thirst, shortness of breath, weakness, lack of appetite, chilling, pallor of the face, bluish lips and nails, and dizziness. Headache is also very common and may be quite severe. A very forceful pounding of the heart may be noted as if exercising strenuously although the individual may, in fact, not consider himself doing so.

The first aid is to either administer more oxygen or to allow the individual time to acclimatize so that he requires less. This essentially limits the first aider to only a few choices:

1. Administer oxygen from containers which is usually impractical and seldom done at altitude (with the exception of climbing above 22,000 feet).

2. Descend to lower altitude.

3. Make a conscious effort to breathe deeper or faster, thereby getting more oxygen into the system. This, however, can be tiring and occasionally if carried too far can produce dizziness or even nausea due to excessive loss of carbon dioxide.

4. Slow down, utilizing the "rest step" if needed, thereby reducing the body's need for oxygen.

For most who are reasonably acclimatized, the last two choices are adequate. There are occasions, however, when individuals are forced to descend to lower altitudes because of "acute" mountain sickness. As first aiders, do not hesitate to suggest this rather than encouraging the individual to go beyond a reasonable level of discomfort.

After arriving at high altitude, rest is essential. Only light physical exertion should be performed for the first 24 hours.

Pulmonary edema

Pulmonary edema is the leakage of blood plasma into the lungs, thereby rendering the air sacs (alveoli) ineffective for exchanging oxygen and carbon dioxide. The exact manner in which this occurs is not fully understood. There are several characteristics of the problem, however, that have been identified.

1. Pulmonary edema appears to be triggered by the body's response to oxygen deficiency. It occurs most often above 9,000 feet, the average in the United States being about 12,000 feet.

2. It takes from 12 to 36 hours after oxygen deficiency begins before its symptoms appear.

3. The greater the exertion at altitude, the more likely is the development of edema. Conversely, the likelihood is decreased by rest.

4. Serious problems occur in less than one per cent of the climbing population. Once one has had pulmonary edema, however, the chance of its reoccurrence is increased.

5. Various drugs taken for acclimatization may or may not help. Their benefits and risks are not fully defined.

The early symptoms of pulmonary edema are similar to those of acute mountain sickness: extreme weakness, shortness of breath or "tightness" in the chest, nausea, vomiting, a dry cough which progresses to a moist crackling sound, blood in the sputum, very rapid pulse (120 to 160 per minute), "noisy" breathing (bubbling sounds in the chest) and cyanosis of the fingernails, face and lips.

If the symptoms are allowed to continue, the victim will rapidly move into the final phase characterized by unconsciousness and possibly frothy clear or pink bubbles in the mouth or nose. If the unconscious victim is not immediately moved to lower elevations or does not receive oxygen, he will die. All of the early symptoms may be mistaken for "mountain sickness" or fatigue or may pass unnoticed during the night with the morning finding the victim unconscious in the final phase. The final stage of death from hypothermia may be mistaken for pulmonary edema.

By far the best prevention is to climb slowly. Above 10,000 feet, it is wise to take at least one day to acclimatize. At the first sign of mental confusion, severe headache or excessive coughing, the climber should be evacuated to lower altitude as rapidly as possible.

other emergencies

Heart emergencies

Many people fear that any pain or discomfort above the heart or anywhere in the chest is a sign of a seriously ailing heart. Such fear is largely unfounded. There are many conditions not related to the heart that can cause pain or discomfort in the chest. Among these are disorders of various parts of the gastro-intestinal tract, pain in the nerves that lie along the ribs, rib fractures, arthritis involving the joints of the back and ribs, and pneumonia or other conditions involving the lungs. The important point to remember is that only a physician can determine the cause and the degree of seriousness of pain or discomfort in the chest. Several kinds of heart conditions can occur.

Heart attack (coronary thrombosis) is a blockage in a coronary artery which deprives a portion of the heart muscle of normally oxygenated blood. If the deprivation continues, this portion of the heart muscle dies. Typically victims have severe pain, usually described as a crushing pressure beneath the breast bone (sternum), a feeling of apprehension, shortness of breath, vomiting or nausea, and sweating. The pain may appear first in the left arm, move into the neck and then to the left side of the chest. The pain is usually excruciating, vise-like and steady, but may be milder and is sometimes misinterpreted as indigestion.

Another type of heart condition frequently encountered is **angina pectoris**, or chest pain. It is caused by a decreased blood supply to the heart muscle because of a narrowing of a coronary artery. This decreased flow causes periodically recurring pain which is similar to that of a heart attack, although it is usually not as intense. Usually precipated by emotional stress, physical effort, or exposure to cold, it is generally relieved by rest and may last less than five minutes.

In cases of **heart failure,** the heart is no longer able to pump adequately and gradually weakens. Symptoms may include:

1. Shortness of breath, at first on exertion, but later even at rest.
2. Swelling of the feet and ankles.
3. The lips, fingertips, ear lobes and sometimes the face may appear blue.
4. Breathing may be noisy, wheezing and accompanied by coughing, perhaps with blood in the sputum.

68

5. The victim may find it difficult to lie flat.

6. Weakness, dizziness or faintness may be present.

7. The skin may be cold and clammy.

The treatment of victims with all types of heart conditions is basically the same:

1. Place the victim in a comfortable position either lying down or sitting.

2. Administer oxygen if available.

3. Provide comfort and reassurance.

4. Assist in the adminstration of the victim's prescription medicine at his request, carefully noting the time it was given and what it is.

5. Do not allow the victim to move or be immediately transported since exertion or movement puts an additional burden on the heart.

Diabetic coma and insulin shock

Diabetics should identify themselves to the party leader before the trip is begun since two conditions could possibly occur: diabetic coma or insulin shock. The causes, symptoms, and first aid for each are quite distinct. In summary, they are:

	Diabetic coma	Insulin shock
Causes:		
Carbohydrate Intake	Excessive	
Insulin		Excessive
Signs and Symptoms:		
Onset	Gradual —— days	Sudden —— minutes
Skin	Red and dry	Moist and pale
Mouth	Dry	Drooling
Thirst	Intense	Absent
Vomiting	Common	Uncommon
Abdominal Pain	Frequent	Absent
Breath	Acetone odor	No odor
Vision	Dim	Double
Pulse	Weak and rapid	Full and rapid
Convulsions	None	In later stages
Improvement	Gradual — 6-12 hours	Rapid
First Aid:	Administration of insulin	Administration of carbohydrates

If the first aider is still in doubt as to whether the victim is in a diabetic coma or insulin shock, sugar should be administered. In this case, if the victim is in insulin shock, brain damage or death can be prevented. If the victim is in a diabetic coma (too much sugar), there is little risk of seriously worsening the situation. If there is no immediate improvement, a diabetic coma can be diagnosed and the victim promptly evacuated. If the victim is unconscious or is unable to swallow, sugar should be placed under the tongue. It will be absorbed into the blood stream through the lining of the mouth.

Apoplexy

Apoplexy, or stroke, refers to a condition in which a portion of the brain suddenly loses its function due to inadequate blood supply. This usually results from a spontaneous rupture of a blood vessel or the formation of a blood clot that interferes with circulation. If damage is severe, death may occur.

Symptoms usually occur suddenly and dramatically. They include unconsciousness, confusion or dizziness, paralysis or numbness on one side of the body, pupils unequal in size, lack of ability to talk or slurring of speech, convulsions, and loss of bladder and bowel control.

First aid is primarily confined to keeping the victim quiet. Give nothing by mouth and provide oxygen if available. Obtaining medical help is a top priority.

Snake bites

Snake bites are not uncommon in many areas in the United States. Assuming the snake is poisonous, its victim will appear nauseous, weak, dizzy, short of breath, and may even lapse into unconsciousness. These signs may appear quickly or may take an hour or more.

If they do appear, or if the snake is identified as being poisonous:

1. Have the victim stop muscular activity. Violent exercise circulates the venom more rapidly.

2. Tie a CONSTRICTING band firmly above the bite. NOTE the word is "constricting," NOT "tourniquet." The object is to restrict the returning venous blood, NOT the arterial blood. A pulse must be present beyond the site of the constriction.

3. If less than one-half hour has passed since the bite, sterilize a razor blade in a flame. Make a shallow (1/16 to $\frac{1}{8}$ inch) lengthwise incision, $\frac{1}{4}$ to $\frac{3}{8}$ inch long, through each fang mark.

4. Apply suction with the mouth for from 30 minutes to an hour. The venom will cause no harm to the person doing this if he does not swallow it or have an open wound in the mouth.

5. Do not apply cold packs. This inhibits the body's natural enzymes from detoxifying the venom, and does not significantly inhibit the venom from spreading.

6. Lower the injury site to a position below the heart, if possible, to help reduce circulation.

miscellaneous miseries

Blisters

Blisters are most often caused by friction, such as that produced by a loose shoe or poorly fitting pack strap. If detected in the early stages of development, the tender area may be covered with adhesive tape or "moleskin" to prevent the formation of a blister. If a blister has already formed, it may be protected by applying "molefoam" around but not on it, thereby protecting the area yet keeping pressure off it. Cutting a hole in the center of the pad is one method of providing such protection.

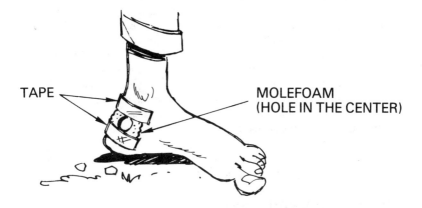

TAPE

MOLEFOAM
(HOLE IN THE CENTER)

Because of the risk of infection, blisters should not be opened unless absolutely necessary. If it must be done, wash the area with soap and water and insert a needle sterilized with a match under the blister's edge. Gently press out the fluid and apply a sterile bandage. If the blister has already broken, it should be washed and bandaged in the same manner and carefully watched for subsequent infection.

Headache

Headache in the mountains usually results from inadequate sunglasses, lack of oxygen, tension in neck muscles, constipation, or some pre-existing physical condition. An occasional cause is swelling of the brain tissue, when over a period of several days a person has sweated excessively and consumed great quantities of water without taking salt tablets. In any case of headache, the source of the trouble should be sought and eliminated by better protection of head or eyes, stretching and relaxing neck muscles, salt tablets, or a laxative. Aspirin relieves the immediate pain.

Nosebleeds

Nosebleeds are quite common and most, minor in nature, are caused by a sudden force, changes in elevation, activity, cold, etc. Direct pressure firmly against the nostril or clamping the tip of the nose is usually sufficient to cause coagulation and stoppage of bleeding. A sitting position with the head slightly tilted back, but not far enough to cause blood to drain back into the throat, or a supine position with the head and shoulders raised, is recommended. Cold applications to the nose may also help.

Fainting

Fainting is a condition in which there is a temporary inadequacy of the circulatory system resulting in a reduced blood supply to the brain. The condition occurs as a result of standing for long periods, getting up suddenly after resting, exercising rapidly after rest, or, rarely, from fright.

Recovery is rapid once the individual is laid down, allowing blood to be circulated into the head. Should recovery not be rapid (within a few minutes), a more serious problem should be considered such as insulin reaction, epileptic seizure, head injury, illness or disease, heart attack, apoplexy, hypothermia, heat stroke, drugs, intoxication, heat exhaustion, suffocation, or electric shock, depending on the supporting history and circumstances.

If a party member feels faint, he should sit down with his head between his knees, or preferably, lie down until he feels better.

Insect bites and stings

No discussion of common emergencies would be complete without a few words about our insect and reptile friends, whose size and ferocity are only surpassed by the imaginations of their victims.

There are, on the market, many commercial insect repellents with varying degrees of effectiveness. Spray and liquid applications seem to provide the best protection in that order. The most effective contain high percentages of N,N - Diethyl-meta-Tolmamide. Products like Off, 410 and Cutter appear quite good. Regardless of the brand and its effectiveness, however, an individual will be bitten occasionally.

If a tick has lodged on the skin and has not yet burrowed in, it may be gently and carefully removed by pulling. If this is not successful or if the tick has lodged under the skin, the best method of removal is to cover it with cooking oil or margarine, thereby closing its breathing pores. If oil or margarine is not available, hot soapy water may be used. Often the tick will back out within a few minutes. If not, again try gentle pulling. If any portion of the body separates and remains imbedded, cleanse the area, cover and seek medical assistance.

Bee stings can be quite serious, particularly for those individuals who have allergic reactions. In fact, more people die of bee stings annually in the United States than from snake bites. Fortunately, however, most individuals who are allergic are aware of their problem and carry prescription medicine. To others, bee stings are normally only a mildly painful and annoying experience which can be reduced by the immediate application of ice or ice water. The stinger should be removed if at all possible.

victim examination

Examination of the victim is one of the most important and fundamental skills which the first aider must develop. Before proper emergency care can be administered, the first aider must determine the extent of the injuries or nature of the illness. Without doing that, he is helpless in assisting the victim. VICTIM EXAMINATION IS THE AREA IN WHICH ALL PREVIOUS TRAINING IS BROUGHT TOGETHER—SIFTED TO DETERMINE THE TWO OR THREE POSSIBLE CAUSES OF DISTRESS AND THE PROPER ACTION APPLIED.

Examination and evaluation of signs and symptoms

There are two levels of victim examination. First a **rapid evaluation** of the victim's overall condition to determine the requirements for urgently needed first aid. The first aider must quickly determine if the victim's respiration or circulation has stopped or if he is bleeding severely. He must take care of these urgent first aid problems immediately without bothering with further prolonged examination. He must not be fooled into checking for only one problem while neglecting the others. This step can be completed in seconds.

The second examination is more complete, in fact **very complete.** Time is normally not a significant factor. It would be disastrous to discover only after placing a bandage on a cut forehead that the victim additionally suffered a fractured cervical vertebra which damaged the spinal cord when the head was moved during bandaging. REMEMBER: NEVER assume that the obvious injuries are the only ones present, nor that they are necessarily the most important. A thorough examination should be conducted in the same careful manner as in determining if the individual is breathing and if his blood is circulating. That is:

Feel: the strength and rate of pulse, the skin temperature, and to find bleeding and unusual bumps or deformities.

Look: at the depth and rate of respiration, at the eyes, at the extent of injuries, at the skin color, and for telltale signs of drugs, alcohol, or medical identification bracelet or tag.

Listen: to what the victim has to say about where it hurts, how it happened, whether it has occurred before, and to judge his level of consciousness.

A tremendous amount of information can be obtained by **asking the victim questions** about his problem. For example, if he complains of pain, ask: Where does it hurt? (if it is not obvious) How was the injury caused? If the injury was not caused by a fall or blow, has the victim had the pain before? If not, did the victim take anything internally, or fail to take something internally he should have (salt tablets, sugar) or did he cause the body to respond in some abnormal way by outside activity (overexertion, high altitude, etc.)? Continue questioning until very rapidly a reasonable assessment of the situation can be made.

Simultaneously, the first aider conducts a comprehensive head-to-toe physical examination proceeding in the following manner:

1. **Check the head.** Run your ha.ids through the hair, feeling for any bumps, indentations or bleeding. Begin at the back of the neck and work to the top of the head in the direction traction would be applied if an injury to the neck existed. If blood is present, separate the hair strands carefully to determine the extent of the injury. DO NOT MOVE THE HEAD while checking for scalp wounds.

   Examine the ears and nose to determine if there is any cerebrospinal fluid or bleeding present. Make a careful distinction between the two. Examine the mouth inside and out, and movements of facial expressions. Ask yourself if the victim's facial expressions are normal. Examine the victim's eyes to determine if the pupils are dilated or constricted, equal in size, and respond to light. Determine if the eyes are synchronized from side to side and up and down. Be thorough and comprehensive.

2. **Check the spine.** Look and feel gently for deformity or boney protrusions in the neck. Notice if the head is positioned in an abnormal manner. If it is, DO NOT ATTEMPT TO STRAIGHTEN but splint as is. Run your hands gently under the back and along the spinal column to identify points of tenderness, pain, or bleeding. If you identify something suspicious, STOP, ASSUME THE WORST, and investigate in more detail for signs of spinal cord injury.

3. **Check the chest.** Look to see if the chest is rising and falling in a normal manner, i.e., both sides are rising together. Gently feel the chest cage for tenderness over fractured or bruised ribs. Feel for depressions indicating crushed ribs, or a grating feeling caused by movement of the broken rib ends against each other.

4. **Check the abdomen.** Gently press against the abdomen. If it is extremely hard or in spasm, this indicates possible internal bleeding or a condition in which the contents of the internal organs have spilled into the abdominal cavity.

5. **Check the pelvic area.** Gently compress the pelvic girth and then press downward to identify grating or tenderness. Check for the characteristic abnormal rolling outward of the leg indicating a fractured hip.

6. **Check upper and lower extremities.** Examine for swelling, discoloration, lumps and tenderness associated with a fracture. Look for unusual or abnormal deformity. Next, if no fractures are evident, check to determine if there is any paralysis (indicating spinal cord damage). Ask the victim if he has any sensation in his arms and legs. If he can respond by raising his arms or legs against the resistance of the examiner's hand, he probably does not have any spinal cord damage. If, on the other hand, he complains of numbness or a tingling sensation, one should suspect spinal damage and treat accordingly. Be as detailed as possible. If the victim complains of numbness or tingling in an arm or leg, determine if the other is normal. Again, assuming no fractures, have him raise his arms. Ask him to grip your hand and squeeze, double checking the extent of the suspected injury as being the upper spinal cord (vs. paralysis of the legs indicating a lower spinal fracture).

7. **Check the buttocks.** Carefully feel underneath the individual for irregularities and bleeding that might not be obvious if the individual is on his back. If the victim is conscious, and no spinal damage is evident, roll the victim slightly onto one side, if required, to ensure a complete examination.

Now that you are satisfied you know what the injuries are, you are ready to perform first aid.

If the victim is unconscious, or semi-conscious so as not to be a help, diagnosis is severely complicated. In that case, one must utilize external signs and symptoms alone to determine the problem.

The first aider must be aware of other basic diagnostic signs and techniques used to rapidly assess a probable injury or illness to perform necessary first aid. One useful technique, for example, is to compare the victim's condition with a "normal" individual. (It is realized that "normal" versus "abnormal" are not precise terms since they depend upon age, sex, physical condition, fatigue, mental state, etc., but, for our purposes, they fit.) There are seven general conditions that can be observed:

Physiological signs	Normal values
Respiration	12-15 breaths per minute in adults 20 breaths per minute in children
Pulse	60-80 in adults 80-100 in children 120 in infants
Skin color and temperature	Pink and warm (98.6°F)
Pupils of the eyes	Regular in outline and of the same size Contract upon exposure to light
Sensation to pain	Reacts to physical stimuli
State of consciousness	Fully alert, oriented and responsive to vocal or physical stimuli
Ability to move	Easily upon command

Obviously, when an unconscious person is being examined, ability to move cannot be compared. State of consciousness can subjectively be determined by noting the level of response to physical surroundings. Some, although unconscious, respond to their name verbally, or moan randomly, or react to pain loudly, etc., indicating roughly the extent of the immediate injury. Even though an individual is unconscious, too, he will respond to pain stimuli, such as the pricking of the skin with a pin, by triggering an involuntary muscular reaction thereby forcing an extremity to jump or withdraw. Other physiological signs can readily be checked with reasonable assurance that their values can be used in predicting the injury or illness.

After the first aider has compared the victim's physiological signs with normality, he must next identify all possible reasons why that individual is unconscious. In the following chapters it will become obvious that in the backcountry the first aider may not want to allow the unconscious victim to lie there until help arrives. His condition may require immediate evacuation, oxygen, special drugs, or special methods of evacuation.

The possibilities causing an individual to become unconscious or semi-conscious then, include the following, although the list is not comprehensive:

1. EXTERNAL causes such as: lightning, excess heat or cold, lack of oxygen and poisoning, which lead to electrical shock, heat exhaustion, heat stroke, hypothermia, pulmonary edema,

asphyxia, suffocation, drug and alcohol problems, drowning and dehydration.

2. INTERNAL DISORDERS such as: heart attack, diabetic coma, insulin shock, fever illness and apoplexy.

3. TEMPORARY CONDITIONS such as: fainting or physical exhaustion.

4. INJURY such as: head injury, loss of blood, shock, etc.

If the first aider knows the signs and symptoms of these, he can then make a comparison that will readily identify a set of probable causes of the problem. This process is displayed graphically on the following page. As the first aider evaluates, he must take notes on his findings, suspected reasons for the unconsciousness and on the victim's condition as it changes over a period of time. In cases of shock, for example, the victim's condition can be identified and improvement observed by the regular observation of pulse, respiration, skin color and temperature.

Questions of circumstance

Finally, the first aider has one additional set of clues at his disposal besides a comparison of signs and symptoms. He has a set of "questions of circumstance" which give an immediate positive indication of the problem before he needs to make any comparisons. The first aider, will, for example, ask questions of himself and others around, such as:

Is there any physical injury — shock, head injury, bleeding?

What are the weather and other external conditions—heat, cold, high altitude, lightning? Could any of these have contributed to the victim's condition?

Has the victim taken anything internally—alcohol, drugs, medication, insulin?

Is the individual under medication or has he been sick—nitroglycerin, cold pills, ill, disease?

Is there anything unusual in his belongings or on his person—medical alert tag, medication, drugs, etc.?

When was the last time the individual ate or drank relative to the amount of physical activity? Could he be suffering from heat exhaustion, dehydration or physical collapse?

Did the victim complain or act unusual before he collapsed, possibly indicating heart attack, physical exhaustion, apoplexy, seizure or insulin shock?

SIGNS AND SYMPTOMS RELATED TO CAUSES OF UNCONSCIOUSNESS

Respiration
- Shallow — Intoxication, drugs, head injury, shock, fainting, heat exhaustion, insulin shock, electric shock, hypothermia, poisoning.
- Shortness of Breath — Heart attack, pulmonary edema, physical exhaustion.
- Normal — Poisons, illness, insulin shock.
- Labored — Heat stroke, apoplexy, airway obstruction, heart failure.
- Irregular — Shock, fainting, hypothermia, poison, epilepsy.
- Deep — Apoplexy, intoxication, drugs, head injury, diabetic coma, heart failure.
- Slow — Hypothermia, drugs, intoxication.

Pulse
- Strong and Rapid — Heat stroke, intoxication, drugs, insulin shock.
- Strong and Slow — Apoplexy, intoxication, drugs, head injury.
- Weak and Rapid — Heart attack, drugs, head injury, diabetic coma, shock, heat exhaustion, pulmonary edema, physical exhaustion, apoplexy.
- Weak and Slow — Intoxication, drugs, fainting, hypothermia, electric shock.
- Irregular — Heart attack, drugs, hypothermia.

Skin

Temperature
- Hot — Heat stroke, diabetic coma, high fever.
- Normal — Apoplexy, intoxication, drugs, head injury, heat exhaustion, pulmonary edema.
- Cold — Apoplexy, drugs, intoxication, head injury, shock, heat exhaustion, fainting, hypothermia, asphyxia, suffocation, electric shock, physical exhaustion.

Moistness
- Dry — Heat stroke, diabetic coma, high fever.
- Normal — Head injury, intoxication, drugs, apoplexy.
- Moist — Head injury, intoxication, drugs, apoplexy, shock, heat exhaustion, fainting, insulin shock, suffocation, electric shock.

Color
- Red — Heat stroke, apoplexy, intoxication, drugs, head injury, epilepsy, diabetic coma, carbon monoxide poisoning.
- Normal — Apoplexy, intoxication, drugs, head injury, epilepsy.
- Pale - Apoplexy, intoxication, drugs, head injury, epilepsy, shock, heat exhaustion, fainting, insulin shock, hypothermia, suffocation, asphyxia, illness, pulmonary edema, physical exhaustion, heart attack.

Pupils
- Normal — Intoxication, drugs, shock, heat exhaustion, fainting, insulin shock, suffocation.
- Unequal — Apoplexy, head injury.
- Constricted — Head injury, drug use.
- Dilated — Heat stroke, intoxication, drugs, shock, heat exhaustion, fainting, insulin shock, suffocation, electric shock, apoplexy, heart attack, hypothermia, head injury, epilepsy.

Other Signs
- Alcohol on Breath — Intoxication.
- Physical Weakness — Heat exhaustion, fainting, poison, physical exhaustion, pulmonary edema.
- Headache, Nausea — Sunstroke, shock, heat exhaustion, poison, head injury.
- Paralysis, Twitching — Stroke, convulsions, epilepsy, head injury.
- Acetone Odor Breath — Diabetic coma, hypothermia.
- Restless — Shock, heart attack, convulsions.
- Muscular cramps — Heat exhaustion
- Coughing, Congested Chest — Pulmonary edema.
- Bleeding at nose, ear or mouth — Head injury.
- Acting Unusual or Irrational — Hypothermia, Drugs, Intoxication.

Between **Signs and symptoms** and **Questions of circumstance,** the first aider can usually reasonably identify the set of candidate problems, even in the most difficult situation.

Triage

Sometimes a situation can become extremely complicated when an entire rope team is involved in an accident causing multiple injuries to two or more members. The first aider must then employ a procedure known as triage—the sorting of accident victims according to the severity of their injuries. The reason for triage is simple: If the victims are selected for treatment at random, those with minor injuries may be treated before those with life-threatening problems. A situation the first aider must AVOID is the tendency to provide care to the one who yells the loudest at the expense of the victim who is quietly bleeding to death or suffering respiratory arrest. Another common error is treating the injuries first that appear to be the most serious. As an example, one individual may be covered with blood from a small forehead cut while another, who appears to have only a slight chest pain, actually has a sucking chest wound. The first aider must identify the injuries with enough care to be able to sort the victims into three groups:

High priority injuries
    Airway and breathing difficulties
    Cardiac arrest
    Uncontrolled bleeding
    Severe head injuries
    Penetrating chest injuries or open abdominal wounds
    Severe medical problems
        Poisonings
        Heat stroke
        Illness
Second priority injuries
    Multiple fractures
    Severe burns
    Back injuries
Lowest priority injuries
    Minor fractures
    Minor wounds
    Obviously dead

Only after the victims have been sorted can the first aider start emergency care procedures, obviously treating the high priority injuries first.

drugs

Because of possible harm that can result from the administration of drugs and legal implications, first aiders are allowed ONLY to administer a victim's prescription at his request, and even so, should have a witness present. Under no circumstances should a first aider administer his own prescription drug to the victim even though he may believe it is suitable. The type of drug used, its dosage and method of administration depend upon the victim's symptoms, actual injuries, past medical history, the length of time after the injury before it is administered, and future drugs or anaesthesia to be used once medical help is obtained. If not administered correctly or at the right time, drugs can do more harm than good.

The one exception to the above, when used properly, is aspirin. It is one of the most effective drugs for relieving pain provided that:

1. It is not used in circumstances which might mask the fever of an infection before that possibility has been realized.
2. The victim is not allergic to it.
3. Excessive quanitities are not consumed. Aspirin IS the most common cause of poisoning in young children. The normal adult dosage is two 0.6 gram tablets orally every 4 hours.

Regrettably, drug abuse is becoming more prevalent, particularly in the outdoors. A general knowledge of various drug symptoms and the first aid for overdose victims, therefore, is essential.

ABOUT DRUGS

Drug	Pharmacologic classification	Physical symptoms and behavior patterns	Major dangers	First aid
Narcotics: Opium, Morphine, Heroin, Codeine, Paregoric, Synthetic Narcotics (Demerol-Methadone)	Central nervous system depressants	Reactions to drug: reduction of pain, lessening of anxiety and tension, decreased activity, lethargy, decrease in breathing and pulse rate, pinpoint pupils, muscle relaxation, profuse sweating, decrease in body temperature, dizziness, nausea, vomiting, constipation. Withdrawal symptoms: nervousness, restlessness, anxiety, sweating, hot and cold flashes, nausea, vomiting, diarrhea, dilated pupils, increased respiration, blood pressure and body temperature.	General physical deterioration, anti-social acts, interference of pain threshhold. Painful withdrawal symptoms. Death from overdose.	Arouse the victim. Keep him on his feet. Maintain an open airway. Give artificial respiration if necessary. Reassure victim.
Barbiturates (Sleeping Pills) Luminal, Nembutal, Amytal, Seconal	Central nervous system depressants	Relief of anxiety, contentment, constricted pupils, drunk appearance, slurred speech, incoherency, depression, drowsiness, dullness, unconsciousness.	May cause damage to brain or liver. Some indication of kidney damage. Painful withdrawal symptoms. Pneumonia, convulsions. Death from overdose.	Maintain open airway. Give artificial respiration if necessary. Maintain body temperature.

Drug	Pharmacologic classification	Physical symptoms and behavior patterns	Major dangers	First aid
Amphetamines: (Pep Pills) Benzedrine, Dexedrine, Methedrine, Methamphetamine	Central nervous system stimulants	Rapid speech, alertness, relief from fatigue, confused thinking, excitability, sleeplessness, nervousness, irritability, fear, hallucinations, aggressive behavior.	Malnutrition, exhaustion, pneumonia, delusions and deliriums. Can develop high blood pressure or heart attacks. Effects on circulatory system. Potential brain damage.	Protect victim. Maintain open airway. Give artificail respiration if necessary. Maintain body temperature.
Cocaine	Central nervous system stimulant	Dilated pupils, loss of appetite-weight, euphoria, feelings of well-being, excitability, restlessness, tremors, especially of hands.	Mental confusion and dizziness, depression, feelings of persecution, and convulsions. Death from overdose.	Protect victim. Maintain open airway. Give artificial respiration if necessary. Maintain body temperature.
Hallucinogens: LSD (Psychedelics) Mescaline	Central nervous system stimulants and/or depressants	Dilated pupils, cold hands and feet, goose pimples, nausea, vomiting, chills, trembling, illusions, delusions, hallucinations, laughing, crying, anxiety, incoherent speech, increased heart beat and blood pressure, increase in body temperature and flushed face.	Bizarre mental effects, unpredictable behavior. Exhibits dangerous acts of invulnerability. Chromosomal damage. Possible brain damage. Suicidal tendencies.	Reassure and protect from bodily harm.
Marihuana (Common term for Canabis sativa)	Central nervous system stimulant and/or depressant Hallucinogen	Reddening of eyes. Dry mouth-throat, increased heart rate, increase of appetite. Coughing spells. Euphoria, exaggerated sensory perceptions. Talkative-laughter. Drunk appearance.	May hinder physical and mental functions. Distortion in sense perceptions, especially time and space. Can facilitate contact with persons using more dangerous drugs. Interferes with pain threshhold. Psychotic effects may develop.	None required.

83

Drug	Pharmacologic classification	Physical symptoms and behavior patterns	Major dangers	First aid
Tranquilizers: Major Phenothiazines Valium Minor Equanil Librium	Central nervous system depressants	Sleep producing, nausea, vomiting, depression, mental sluggishness, urinary retention, constipation, slurred speech, unconsciousness, fall in body temperature and blood pressure.	Visual disturbances, dizziness, hyperexcited, hazardous irrational acts, drowsiness, interferes with pain threshhold.	Arouse the victim. Maintain open airways. Give artificial respiration if necessary. Maintain body temperature.
Deliriants: (violatile chemical compounds used in sniffing) Airplane glue, plastic cement, Toluene, paint thinners, gasoline, Freon	Central nervous system depressants	Initial excitement, enlarged eye pupils, double vision, excessive oral secretion, irritation around the nose and mouth, sneezing, coughing, chest pain, hearing difficulties, drunk appearance. Angry, irritable, drowsiness, unconsciousness.	Bizarre mental effects, anti-social acts. May exhibit dangerous acts of invulnerability. Long and heavy use has potential for serious damage to brain, heart, lungs, kidney, liver and other organs. Death from choking or suffocation.	Maintain open airway. Give artificial respiration if necessary. Maintain body temperature.
Alcohol: (Ethyl)	Central nervous system depressant	Drowsiness, offensive odor, incoordination, disturbance of speech, altered respiration, signs of shock, rapid thready pulse, violent, noisy, belligerent, unconsciousness.	Anti-social acts. Danger of self-destruction or injury to oneself or others. Interference with pain threshhold. Irreversible brain and other organ damage, especially to liver. Coma, shock, circulatory and respiratory failure resulting in death. Many effects consistent with barbiturates.	If sleeping normally, maintain body warmth. If abnormal breathing or unconscious, maintain open airway. Give artificial respiration if necessary.

NOTE: At no time should the first aider endanger himself or the rest of the party. If you cannot control the situation, wait until help arrives.

the mountaineering first aid kit

Mountaineering first aid begins with the first aid kit, an essential which must be carried by every person on every trip. The kit should be small, compact, sturdy, and waterproof; a polyethylene box with a tight lid makes a good container. A metal box which can be used in an emergency to melt snow or warm water is better. The lid is a good place to tape coins for phone calls.

There are dozens of first aid kits on the market—only a small number of which are adequate. There are, also, dozens of lists of recommended contents—again only a few of which are adequate. When selecting a first aid kit, apply the following general guidelines:

1. Ensure there is enough bulk that a significant quantity of blood can be absorbed. In the mountains severe bleeding wounds are a common type of injury and sterile absorbent material cannot be improvised.
2. Stay light but have enough of everything. One small roll of tape and two salt tablets are not a sufficient first aid kit.
3. Consider the area you are traveling into and pack accordingly. If travelling on a glacier for example, where there are no trees and ice axes cannot be spared, and if a member of the party fractures a forearm, a wire splint would be extremely valuable.
4. Avoid carrying drugs unless you are thoroughly familiar with their use. If you feel you need something for your personal use, consult your family physician and let him explain its limitations, dangers and directions for use.

With these thoughts in mind, the following kit is recommended.

THE MOUNTAINEERING FIRST AID KIT

Item	*Quantity and size*	*Use*
Aspirin	12 tablets-5 grain	1 or 2 every 4 hours, for pain
Antacid	6 tablets	For indigestion or heartburn; may be Bucladin, Ulcetral, Rollaids, etc.
Antihistamine	6 tablets	1 every 4 hours for insect bites, colds, or hives
Bandaids	12 1-inch	For lacerations
Butterfly Bandaids (or know how to make)	6 (various sizes)	For closing lacerations
Carlisle (Battle Dressing) or sanitary napkin	1 4-inch	For large bleeding wounds
Moleskin or Molefoam	½ pkg.	For blisters
Needle	1 medium size	To remove splinters, etc.
Tincture of Benzoin	1 oz. bottle (plastic)	To hold tape in place and protect the skin
Antibacterial soap or Tincture of Zepherin	1 oz. bottle (plastic)	Mild antiseptic for abrasions, cuts
Razor blade, single edge or quality scissors	1	For shaving hairy spots before taping
Roller gauze	2 rolls 2" x 5 yd.	For holding gauze flats in place
Safety pins	3 (1 large)	Mending seatless pants
Salt tablets	24	To prevent exhaustion and cramps due to heavy perspiring
Steri-pad gauze flats	6, 4" x 4"	For larger wounds
Cloth tape	2" roll	For sprains, securing dressings, etc.
Triangular bandage	1	For supporting arm, protecting dressing from contamination.

OPTIONAL ITEMS

Drugs	As prescribed by personal physician	If carried, each should be stored in a separate container, and clearly labelled as to dosage, expiration date, type of drug and expected reaction
Elastic bandage	1 3-inch	For securing dressings in place. Training in its use is required
Thermometer	1 (-40°F to 120°F)	For measuring temperature
Wire mesh splint	1	For suspected fractures

Miscellaneous items may include:
2 Dimes and 2 nickels for phone calls in emergencies
First aid/rescue information
Pencil and paper

evacuation

The determination of when to evacuate and whether it should be done by the party or by outside help is a difficult problem. It depends not only upon the condition of the victim but upon the following factors:

1. Number in the party and their condition
2. Location of the party — miles from help
3. Time of day
4. Weather — current and expected
5. Terrain — snow, rock, trail
6. Supplies and experience in the party
7. Reaction time of the help and their technical competence

Obviously, then, the answer to "when" and "by whom" varies drastically from case to case. There are, however, some generalizations that can be made.

When to evacuate

A victim should be evacuated as soon as possible by whatever means available and compatible with his injuries. The longer the delay, the greater the chance of infection and the more difficult surgical repair becomes. His condition, however, should not be compromised in the effort. Since he normally will benefit from a period of rest following the injury, no transportation should be considered until his condition has stabilized. This is best indicated by the victim himself. He should be asked how he feels and his condition closely observed prior to and during transportation. **ONLY UNDER LIFE-THREATENING CONDITIONS CAUSED BY INJURY, WEATHER OR TERRAIN SHOULD EVACUATION BE IMMEDIATE.** In fact, in some injuries, evacuation is best DELAYED until rescue personnel and/or medical assistance is available.

Seldom should the party consider evacuating an injured individual under their own power. The trauma associated with transportation over difficult terrain (including narrow trails) with improvised devices is usually an unnecessary burden on the victim and exhausting to the party. The party saves no time in evacuating a victim off a terraced ridge to a valley floor only to have a helicopter pick him up there. In that instance, the victim's condition is only aggravated, and an additional strain placed on both him and the rest of the party.

There are some exceptions to the above. Evacuation by the party may be considered for injuries that are not major (e.g., a closed fracture of the lower leg or arm), if the accident has occurred near a trail, if the party is strong and sufficiently large (12 or more) to perform the carry adequately, if the distance is less than 3 to 5 miles, AND if the victim's conditions and spirits allow such a move. In other conditions, however, if the accident has occurred in an area requiring technical evacuation (that which requires lowering), where injuries are severe, where distances are extreme OR the party size and/or strength are not sufficient for the carry, evacuation should NOT be attempted. Rather, it is better to wait for assistance. Again, it may not only be easier on the victim, but faster to await possible helicopter pick-up than to attempt evacuation over difficult or lengthy terrain.

EVACUATION SUMMARY CHART

WHEN	UNDER WHAT CONDITIONS
EVACUATE IMMEDIATELY	If victim exhibits symptoms of a major head injury, OR If pulmonary edema is suspected, OR If victim has prolonged unconsciousness, OR If weather or terrain conditions are life-threatening.
DELAY EVACUATION until rescue personnel and/or medical assistance is available	If victim exhibits symptoms of apoplexy, heart attack, internal injuries, neck or spinal fracture, OR of skull fracture.
EVACUATE ROUTINELY BY PARTY	If victim has NOT sustained major injury, AND If party is strong, large, and knowledgeable, AND If the distance to road by trail is less than 3 to 5 miles, AND If the victim's condition is stable and strong.

Evacuation of party members

After it has been decided whether the victim should be evacuated, another question remains: Should some of the remaining members of the party be evacuated? If, for example, some are not prepared for a bivouac situation or have given most of their equipment to the victim, it is better that they leave the accident scene for civilization rather than risk the problems associated with hypothermia, exhaustion, inadequate food consumption, etc. If this decision is made, it is well advised to:

1. Provide first aid, shelter and food to the victim first.

2. Leave the stronger and better equipped members with the victim together with extra food clothing, fuel, etc.

3. Send the remainder of the party down the mountain under suitable leadership before they become victims themselves.

Preparing the victim for evacuation

If it is decided that the victim will require evacuation, regardless of the method, he must be mentally and physically prepared for the move. He should be informed how the evacuation will be conducted and what he should expect. Initially, he should be handled with UNREASONABLY EXTREME CARE until his confidence in the evacuation techniques outweighs his desire to evacuate himself. The first aiders should expect an increase in the victim's pulse, respiration and blood pressure as an indication of his anxiety.

Once mentally prepared, he should be placed into the litter, wrapped in layers of clothing and plastic as appropriate, and securely tied in. It would obviously be disastrous if the victim fell out or even if an arm came undone and was stepped on. It has happened — GUARD AGAINST IT. Place on the victim a pair of goggles and hard hat so that he is reasonably protected. Additionally, conspicuously attach a chronological record of the first aid administered, particularly important if his condition has been unstable, medication given or a tourniquet applied. A duplicate record should always be kept by one of the party members having performed the first aid.

Caring for the victim during evacuation

During evacuation, observe the victim constantly. Talk to him and ask him how he is doing. Stop occasionally to let him rest. For lower extremity injuries, evacuate him with his head downhilll. For chest, head or upper extremity injuries, evacuate him feet first when lowering. Just as in the treatment of shock, carry the victim in a nearly horizontal position when possible, slightly elevating the injured area.

Evacuation by back carry

One method of evacuation, the **back carry,** is particularly good for transporting a victim with minor injuries of the lower or upper extremities short distances to a trail or stretcher. Its limitations are apparent: it is, most obviously, very tiring for the rescuer, and not particularly comfortable for the victim, whose circulation in the lower extremities will be impaired over a period of time.

BACK CARRY

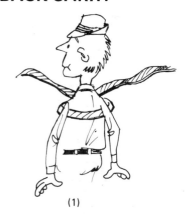

(1)

PASS ONE INCH NYLON
TAPE OR TWO INCH WEBBING
ACROSS THE BACK OF THE
VICTIM UNDER HIS ARMS . . .

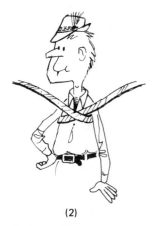

(2)

CROSSING IT IN FRONT OF
HIS CHEST . . .

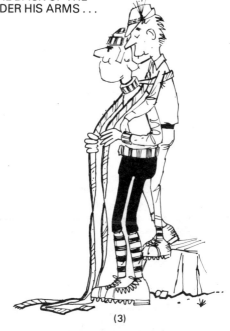

(3)

THEN WITH THE VICTIM AND
RESCUER TOGETHER, PASS THE
WEBBING OVER THE SHOULDERS
OF THE RESCUER . . .

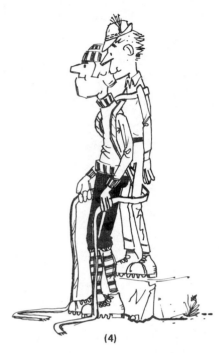

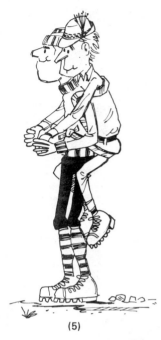

(4)

(5)

THEN AROUND THE VICTIM'S
LEGS ABOVE THE KNEES . . .

WITH THE WEBBING TIED IN A
SQUARE KNOT ACROSS THE
STOMACH OF THE RESCUER
WITH THE ENDS TIED OFF.

If 2-inch webbing is not available, a rope seat may be constructed as an alternative. Construction requires a 120-foot climbing rope coiled into a loop 16 to 20 inches in diameter and secured tightly on one side. The coil is then divided to provide a seat for the victim and shoulder straps for the rescuer. (See following page.)

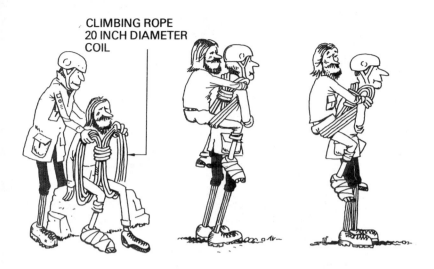

CLIMBING ROPE
20 INCH DIAMETER
COIL

Evacuation by rope stretcher

Another method of evacuation is by a **rope stretcher.** This can be constructed and used with or without the aid of ice axes and/or branches as follows.

Place the rope, preferably 150-foot, extended, on the ground. Find the center. From the center make 16 180° bends, 8 extending on each side of the center. The distance between the bends should be approximately as wide as the victim and the full 16 bends approximately as long as the victim's length. Bring the rope ends around the sides of the stretcher adjacent to the bends. Tie a clove hitch in the rope section adjacent to each bend and insert the bend. Continue tying clove hitches and inserting bends until all the bends are bound. Leave a small loop between the apex of the bend and the knot. Insert the remaining rope through the loops until the entire remainder is coiled around the stretcher. Snug up the knots, tie off the ends and insert padding from the neck to the hips. (See illustration following page.)

Someone should try out the stretcher, whether it is constructed of rope or branches, before placing the victim on it. In this way the need for additional padding or supporting material can be determined without causing discomfort to the victim. CAUTION: evacuation by rope or any improvised stretcher is usually very rough on the victim. If there is a chance that further injury will result, DO NOT EVACUATE until trained rescue personnel with proper equipment are available to assist.

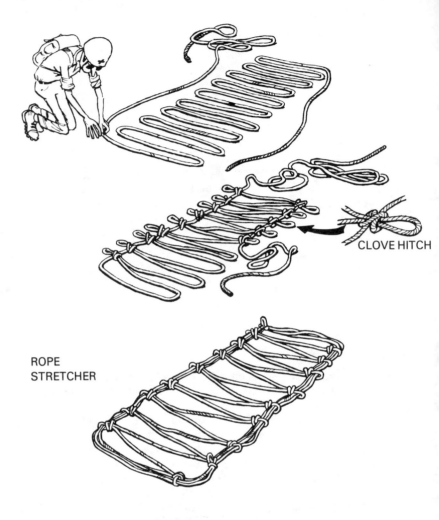

CLOVE HITCH

ROPE
STRETCHER

Evacuation by branch stretcher

Occasionally a situation may arise in which an injury requires immediate evacuation, but outside help is distant. A branch stretcher may be the key to transporting the victim safely and efficiently. It will provide more rigidity than a rope stretcher, is easier to carry, and is more comfortable for the victim.

A branch stretcher must be constructed properly. The following procedures define the MINIMUM requirements for a stretcher capable of transporting an injured victim over about 5 miles of reasonably maintained trail. One may wish to strengthen and reinforce this basic design, but shortcutting it is an invitation to disaster.

94

First, assemble approximately 80 feet of twine, non-stretch cotton or hemp, about ⅛ inch thick. The tensile strength should be about 300 lbs.

To construct the stretcher, cut four poles 8 feet long by 2 inches in diameter and ten smaller poles 2 feet long by 1 inch in diameter. Then, step by step:

1. Position the two long poles and two of the shorter poles to form a rectangle. The short branches should be on top and about a foot in from the ends. They should also extend about 2 inches beyond the edge of the long poles.

2. Position the two other long poles beneath the stretcher diagonally so they cross in the center. These cross poles are needed to make the stretcher rigid and stable.

3. Secure the three pieces at each corner with approximately 8 feet of twine as follows: Double the twine and slip it under the branches. Insert the doubled end through the loop formed by the doubling and tighten back on itself. After one wrap, change direction diagonally crossing the first wrap. Divide the running ends and make two or three opposing turns between the branches and around the twine to tighten it (called frapping), and tie off the ends using a square knot. Be sure all wraps are neat and do not overlap each other. If consecutive wraps overlap, they may later slip over each other, creating slack. Lashing must not be done in a hurry; it takes time to do it properly.

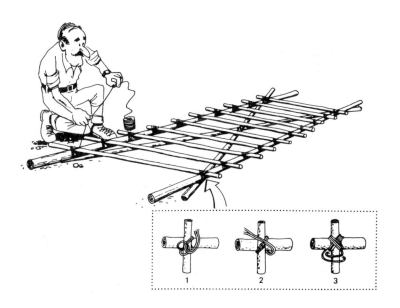

Next, remove all obstacles that could interfere with the aircraft—brush, trees, stumps, and loose rocks and snow, at least 75 feet in diameter of the landing site. If the landing site must be located in an area of soft snow, pack the site and surrounding area to prevent blowing and obstructing the pilot's vision. Make the area as level as possible (within 10 per cent preferred). Clearly mark the landing area with colored tape or other objects of contrasting color. SECURELY ANCHOR ALL OBJECTS with buried 10-pound rocks if necessary. Rotor wash can apprach 60 to 120 mph.

From the air, even brightly colored objects and arm-waving people are barely visible. Consequently, the best method of signalling the helicopter is by smoke grenade (U.S. Coast Guard-approved, available at most marine supply stores). Smoke not only identifies the accident scene and landing site, but tells the pilot wind speed and direction. If a smoke grenade is not available, a small smoky fire can be built well away from the landing area or rotor wash will scatter it for hundreds of feet. As a preferred alternate, use streamers or plastic ribbon located and securely anchored at the edge and downwind from the landing site slightly to the side of the approach pattern. If none of these is available and a fire inappropriate, a party member can stand with arms extended toward the landing site which indicates "Land here. My back is into the wind."

The party also must prepare the victim for transport and perhaps even transport him a short distance to the landing site. Before the helicopter arrives, the victim is informed of what is going to happen and what he should expect—noise, wind and movement. As stated previously, securely tie the victim into the litter. His hands must be restrained to prevent him from reaching and grabbing. Eye and head protection are a must to prevent injury from blowing debris caused by rotor wash. Secure with the victim any gear going with him that the party does not want to carry out, but do not send items (clothing, ropes, etc.) that may be required by the party later. Ensure there are no loose straps, ropes, or clothing. Tag the victim conspicuously with inform. :ion concerning his suspected injuries, the first aid treatment given and his condition. Finally, and most importantly, **do not endanger the victim** by hurrying to ready him for evacuation. If it will take more time to secure him to the stretcher, request the pilot wait, or to return at an appropriate time.

When the helicopter approaches and as the victim is loaded, the following basic Rules of Safety must be followed:

1. If the helicopter lowers a cable with message, radio, or litter, allow it to touch the ground first to dissipate static electricity.

2. If there is a last-minute danger to the helicopter observed by ground personnel, move your arms from the side horizontally to overhead several times indicating "Do Not Land."

3. Keep well away from expected approach and takeoff patterns of the aircraft.

4. Space the remaining short branches at equal distances along the length of the stretcher and secure them with short (2-foot) lengths of twine. These ties, too, are important, since they support the victim and are under load continuously during travel. Each branch should be secured by wrapping the twine around in one direction and then the opposite, forming an x. As before, secure the ends with a square knot.

Completed, the branch stretcher weighs about 35 pounds. Six climbers (minimum) can carry it. Again obviously, before loading the injured victim on, try it out with a volunteer.

Pad the stretcher well, using all available insulative pads and extra clothing. Because the top of the stretcher is elevated, the "log roll" cannot be used to get the victim on the stretcher. Instead, use a seven man hand-lift (three men on each side and one on the head) to raise the victim while an eighth person slides the stretcher under him.

The branch stretcher is intended for trail evacuation only and not for terrain steep enough to require a belay or safety rope. If the terrain is marginal, or if there is any doubt, send for a rigid litter rather than jeopardize the safety or condition of the victim.

Evacuation by helicopter

The helicopter has revolutionized mountain rescue. It has evacuated injured from cliffs and glaciers directly to hospitals quickly and efficiently when by ground it would have taken days of rough and exhausting trravel. It has shown itself, time and again, to make the difference between life and death. Consequently, seldom is evacuation of a victim with improvised stretcher over rough terrain justified. Exceptions are:
1. If the weather is such that a helicopter could not respond.
2. If the victim's injuries are incapacitating but not serious; if there is a large party and the distance is short (3-5 miles by trail).
3. If indications are that the victim's condition is deteriorating or would deteriorate (life-threatening) should he not be promptly evacuated.

In most other instances, therefore, the delay in waiting for helicopter transport is advisable for both speed and comfort.

To prepare for helicopter transportation, the party has much to do. First it must choose and prepare a landing site. The first choice should be an area that gives a 360° approach for landings and takeoffs—i.e., a flat-topped ridge that allows both landings and takeoffs to be made into the wind. If a ridge is not close, then a relatively flat area on a hillside is the next choice where a "drop-off" is possible rather than a "climb-up" during take-offs. The higher the elevation, the less load the helicopter can carry and the more important a drop-off becomes. Choosing a landing site in a valley floor is least desirable.

4. Stay at least 75 feet away from the landing site until the helicopter engine is off and rotor has stopped, or until the pilot signals you to approach. Even after touchdown, the pilot may want to shift the helicopter's position.

5. Always approach or leave the helicopter from the front so the pilot can see you at all times.

6. Never approach or leave the helicopter from any side where the ground is higher than where the helicopter has landed.

7. Keep your head down since the slower the rotor is moving, the lower it will dip (sometimes down to 5 feet).

8. All personnel and especially the victim, should wear hard hats and have eye protection.

9. The victim should not be placed unattended in the helicopter unless he is restrained.

conclusion

It is hoped that the reader has not skipped over sections of this publication. Although it has not been of much use in describing techniques for scaling peaks, getting into physical condition, or easing the weight carried on a 10-day backpack, its intent has been to give the reader meaningful information relevant to the problems he may encounter in the out-of-doors and, more specifically, a greater awareness of the tremendous problems that exist in the event of an accident. Hopefully, this awareness will foster a keener sense of judgment and will stimulate a conscientious effort to prevent, rather than just respond to accidents through: Planning one's own activities, and informing others of their responsibilities by teaching them what they can do. (To do this one does not need to be a professional teacher, only a person interested in informing the outdoor population of the necessity to be prepared.)

REMEMBER: An accident scene is an extremely confused place. It is very difficult to sort through the things that can be done, to identify those which must be done, and then to accomplish them in proper order. Like rock climbing or skiing, it takes practice to become proficient without making mistakes. Without, as a minimum, mentally rehearsing your actions in the event of an accident, you are bound to commit errors that could be fatal.

Therefore, again, it is strongly recommended that your training not be limited to this text. You should round out your first aid education by enrolling in American Red Cross, Industrial, or Bureau of Mines First Aid courses, and your outdoor education by enrolling in any one of a number of well-rounded climbing, hiking or backpacking courses. Additionally, you may find more detailed information on specific topics in the following references.

REFERENCES

American Academy of Orthopedic Surgeons,
Emergency Care and Transportation of the Sick and Injured,
1971.

American Alpine Club,
Accidents in North American Mountaineering,
1973.

American Medical Association,
Standards for Cardiopulmonary Resuscitation (CPR) and Emergency Cardiac Care (ECC),
Journal of the American Medical Association,
February 18, 1974

American Medical Association,
The Wonderful Human Machine,
1971.

American National Red Cross,
Advanced First Aid and Emergency Care,
First Edition, 1973,
Doubleday and Company.

American National Red Cross,
Cardiopulmonary Resuscitation,
1974.

American National Red Cross,
Standard First Aid and Personal Safety,
First Edition, 1973,
Doubleday and Company.

Cooper, Kenneth H., M.D.,
The New Aerobics,
1970.

Dalle-Molle, John,
Helirescue Manual,
published by Washington State Department of Emergency Services, June
1972.

Division of Vocational Education, Ohio State Department of Education,
Emergency Victim Care,
published by Ohio Trade and Industrial Education Service, 1971.

Ferber, Peggy, ed.
Mountaineering: The Freedom of The Hills,
published by The Mountaineers,
Third Edition, 1974.

Grant, Harvey, and Robert Murray,
Emergency Care,
First Edition, 1971.

Lathrop, T.G., M.D.
Hypothermia: Killer of The Unprepared,
published by The Mazamas.

Mariner, Wastl,
Mountain Rescue Techniques,
1963.

Wilkerson, James A., M.D.
Medicine for Mountaineering,
published by The Mountaineers, 1968.
Second Edition, 1975.